MW01040095

The 5-Ingredient
Heart Healthy
Cookbook

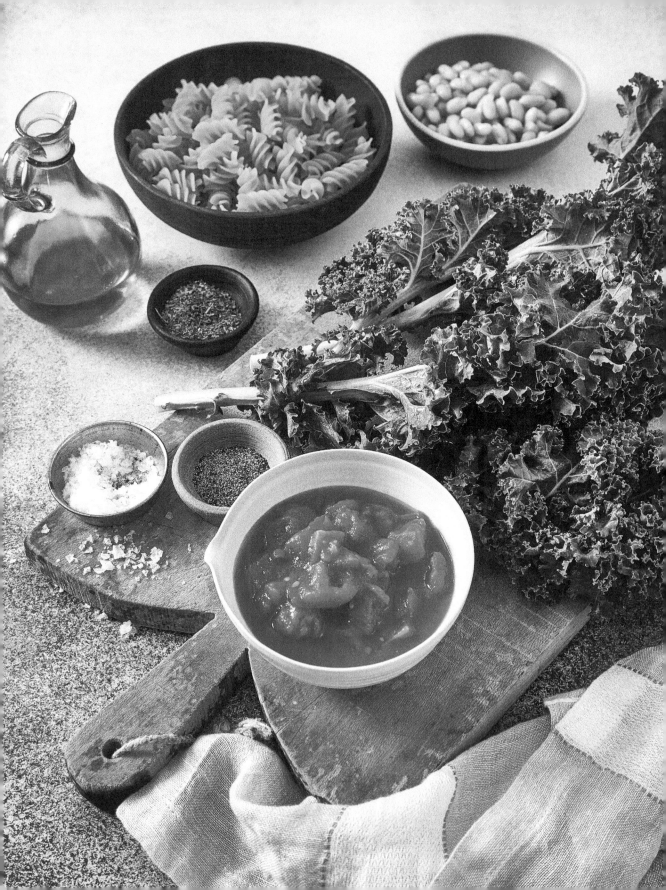

The 5-Ingredient
Heart Healthy Cookbook

101 FLAVORFUL LOW-SODIUM, LOW-FAT RECIPES

Andy De Santis, RD, MPH
and Katherine Green

PHOTOGRAPHY BY HÉLÈNE DUJARDIN

ROCKRIDGE
PRESS

Copyright © 2021 by Rockridge Press, Emeryville, California

No part of this publication may be reproduced, stored in a retrieval system, or transmitted in any form or by any means, electronic, mechanical, photocopying, recording, scanning, or otherwise, except as permitted under Sections 107 or 108 of the 1976 United States Copyright Act, without the prior written permission of the Publisher. Requests to the Publisher for permission should be addressed to the Permissions Department, Rockridge Press, 6005 Shellmound Street, Suite 175, Emeryville, CA 94608.

Limit of Liability/Disclaimer of Warranty: The Publisher and the author make no representations or warranties with respect to the accuracy or completeness of the contents of this work and specifically disclaim all warranties, including without limitation warranties of fitness for a particular purpose. No warranty may be created or extended by sales or promotional materials. The advice and strategies contained herein may not be suitable for every situation. This work is sold with the understanding that the Publisher is not engaged in rendering medical, legal, or other professional advice or services. If professional assistance is required, the services of a competent professional person should be sought. Neither the Publisher nor the author shall be liable for damages arising herefrom. The fact that an individual, organization, or website is referred to in this work as a citation and/or potential source of further information does not mean that the author or the Publisher endorses the information the individual, organization, or website may provide or recommendations they/it may make. Further, readers should be aware that websites listed in this work may have changed or disappeared between when this work was written and when it is read.

For general information on our other products and services or to obtain technical support, please contact our Customer Care Department within the United States at (866) 744-2665, or outside the United States at (510) 253-0500.

Rockridge Press publishes its books in a variety of electronic and print formats. Some content that appears in print may not be available in electronic books, and vice versa.

TRADEMARKS: Rockridge Press and the Rockridge Press logo are trademarks or registered trademarks of Callisto Media Inc. and/or its affiliates, in the United States and other countries, and may not be used without written permission. All other trademarks are the property of their respective owners. Rockridge Press is not associated with any product or vendor mentioned in this book.

Interior and Cover Designer: Monica Cheng
Art Producer: Meg Baggott
Editor: Claire Yee
Production Editor: Ashley Polikoff

Photography © 2020 Hélène Dujardin. Food styling by Anna Hampton.

Author photos courtesy of Natalie CD Photography and Katherine Green.
Cover: Poached Fish in Tomato-Caper Sauce, page 106

ISBN: Print 978-1-64739-974-0
         eBook 978-1-64739-975-7
R0

*To my readers, please know that
your health and happiness are my priority
and that you will find my commitment
to those causes reflected in these pages.*

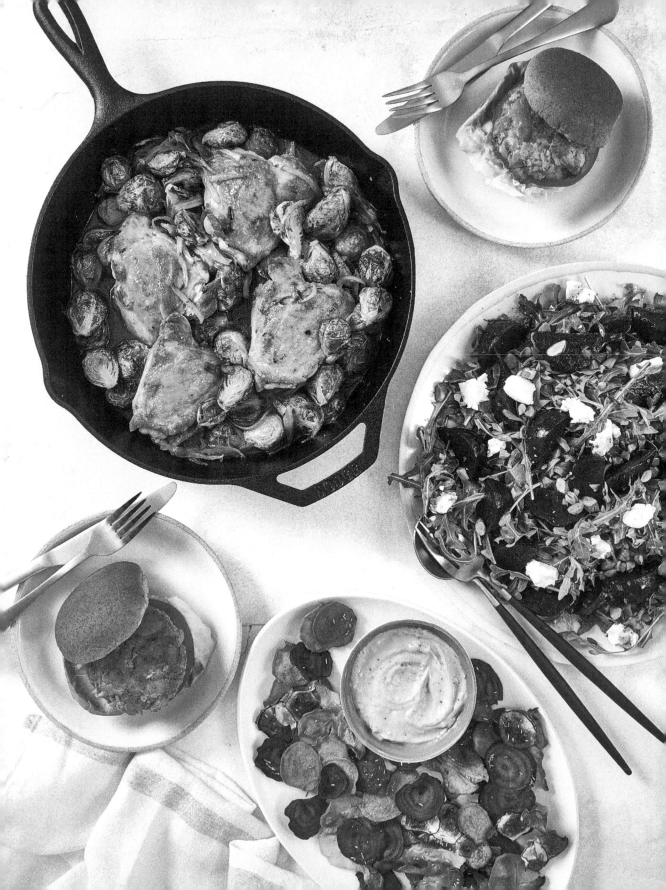

— CONTENTS —

— INTRODUCTION —

Hello everyone, and welcome to *The 5-Ingredient Heart Healthy Cookbook*.

My name is Andy De Santis. I'm a registered dietitian and author from Toronto, Canada, and I'm absolutely thrilled to be guiding you on this journey toward heart-healthy eating. The most important thing that I need you to know about me—aside from the fact that I love kale—is that every single day of the week I help people with goals and challenges similar to your own.

You've probably already consulted friends, family, the internet, and even other health professionals for advice on the topic of heart-healthy eating. I'm willing to bet some of that advice was confusing and conflicting; that's where this book comes in. I fully appreciate that it's not easy to navigate the online nutrition space these days, especially since controversial views are increasingly rewarded with attention even in the absence of good-quality evidence to support them.

In these pages, you can expect guidance that is supported by the best available science yet delivered in a way that is digestible and allows you to understand what you need to do and why you need to do it. Without strictly sticking to one or the other, I will be pulling the best bits of guidance from some of the strongest heart-healthy styles of eating, including Mediterranean, DASH, veganism, and the less well-known but equally effective Portfolio diet pattern.

This advice will be supported by the excellent work of my co-author and recipe developer, Katherine Green, who has done a superb job of bringing my nutrition vision to life with delicious and easy-to-prepare recipes that are practical for use in your daily life and contain only five ingredients per recipe. We want your transition to heart-healthy eating to be as pleasurable as possible, and we're here to support you in the best way we know how. Although this book may not be a replacement for the care and oversight of your primary care team, it's a wonderful complement to their work and a very strong starting point if you are looking to really learn how to use food to take your heart health to the next level.

I can't stress enough just how important nutrition is for your cardiovascular health and longevity. It's the size of the problem and my desire to help as many people as possible fix it that drew me to write this book in the first place. According to the Centers for Disease Control and Prevention (CDC), heart disease is the number-one cause of mortality in the United States and is responsible for nearly one-fourth of the annual deaths, a number that is greater than all types of cancer combined. It's a serious issue and one that I've approached in a very serious manner in this book.

From my vantage point as a private practice dietitian and a writer with an online presence, I do feel that public perception about heart health is at a sort of crossroads. There are more and more personalities, both reputable and otherwise, who are pushing alternative views on the best nutritional practices in this particular area. As I said earlier, my bet is that you've been exposed to some of these views and opinions and may be a bit confused about which eating style really is best for you.

In addition to making your life easier in the kitchen, my primary aim with this book is to make your life easier out of the kitchen, too, by removing some of the confusion and uncertainty around popular heart-health topics, such as fats and cholesterol. I know you're interested in these topics, and I've tried my best to stay current in my approach to make sure you enjoy an authentic written experience with a dietitian, rather than some premade pamphlet you could easily find online. And to save you from having to figure out how to incorporate the information and advice in these pages into actual meals, Katherine and I have made sure that the recipes in this book are based on heart-healthy but affordable and easily accessible ingredients, so you won't struggle to find unusual ingredients or have to search out specialty shops.

And with that I welcome you, once again, to *The 5-Ingredient Heart Healthy Cookbook*.

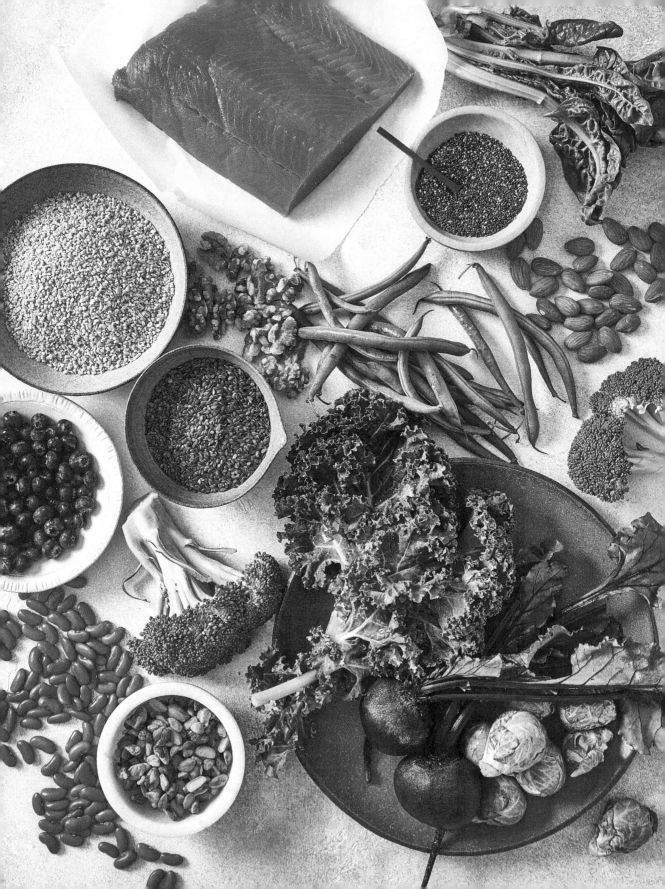

CHAPTER ONE

Heart Health Made Easy

Your heart-health journey begins here, and I'm thrilled to be the one you've chosen to guide you on your path to improved heart health. You can expect a ton of great information in the pages to come.

Not only will I introduce you to my nutrition philosophy as it relates to heart health, but also I will teach you the key groups of foods that will make all the difference going forward. You will leave this chapter with a much greater understanding of not only what to eat but also why certain foods are specifically beneficial to keep your heart working at its best. Although some of these messages may seem obvious to some of you, I promise to throw you a few curveballs while also addressing some of the more controversial topics in this corner of the nutrition world.

I don't want you to feel overwhelmed, though. I appreciate that this style of eating may be new to many of you, but I want you to know that this book will provide all the support and encouragement you need to succeed.

My goal is simply to make your transition into heart-healthier eating as seamless as possible, from our five-ingredient promise to listing the kitchen equipment you will need and everything in between.

Heart health made easy—what could be better? Let's get started.

What Is a Heart-Healthy Diet?

Let's start by defining some of the basic principles associated with the term "heart-healthy diet." This will help us arrive at a mutual understanding before we continue. I'd describe the term primarily as a style of eating that includes as many foods as possible known to directly reduce heart disease risk or reduce the risk factors associated with heart disease, such as high blood pressure, high blood cholesterol, or high blood triglyceride levels. My definition also allows room for foods that you truly enjoy so you can keep your heart healthy and happy in more ways than one.

Depending on personal preferences, this style of eating could look quite different from person to person, but here are some common themes across all heart-healthy diets:

- High in vegetables (especially nonstarchy vegetables) and fruits

- High in traditionally healthy fats such as fish, nuts, seeds, olives, avocado, etc.

- High in plant-based protein sources such as legumes and soy, for those who enjoy them

- High in aquatic protein sources such as fish and seafood

If you've been doing some investigating on your own in the nutrition world, you'll notice that most of these themes are common in many of the popularized heart-health approaches, such as the DASH diet, Mediterranean diet, vegan/vegetarianism, and the lesser-known but equally potent Portfolio diet. Let's take a closer look at these diets.

DASH Diet

The DASH diet, which stands for Dietary Approaches to Stop Hypertension, was developed by the National Institutes of Health in the 1990s to create a style of eating that could fight back against the rise of high blood pressure caused by excessive sodium intake. The DASH style of eating is diverse and inclusive of many different food groups while uniquely emphasizing limits to your daily sodium intake and stressing ample amounts of nutrients associated with lowering blood pressure, such as potassium, calcium, and magnesium.

Mediterranean Diet

In the Mediterranean diet, poultry, dairy, eggs, and red meat are consumed infrequently in order to make way for more whole grains, legumes, fruits, vegetables, fish, and other seafoods. A robust study published in *The New England Journal of Medicine* in 2018 found that for people with a high risk of cardiovascular disease, following a Mediterranean diet reduced the chance of heart attack or stroke.

Vegan/Vegetarian Diet

Probably best characterized as a slightly stricter version of the Mediterranean diet, vegan and vegetarian diets are strongly associated with good heart health. When planned appropriately, they contain a large amount of fiber, vitamins, minerals, and antioxidants.

In 2016, the Academy of Nutrition and Dietetics firmly stated that vegans and vegetarians are at reduced risk of heart disease, hypertension, type 2 diabetes, and certain types of cancer owing to a diet that tends to be high in fruits, vegetables, legumes, soy, nuts, seeds, and whole grains.

Portfolio Diet

I'm strongly connected to the Portfolio diet not only because it is proven to lower cholesterol as laid out in a 2011 study in the *Journal of the American Medical Association*, but also because it was developed in my hometown of Toronto by a clinician scientist named David Jenkins. The Portfolio diet is among the most effective approaches for lowering LDL ("bad" cholesterol levels) and focuses on the inclusion of tree nuts, soy-based foods, and soluble fiber–rich foods such as oatmeal, legumes, and certain types of fruits and vegetables, such as zucchini, sweet potatoes, green beans, kiwi, and strawberries.

As you can see, each of these styles of eating overlaps on some key foods and messages but also possesses unique characteristics. I've taken all of this into account in assembling the heart-healthy eating philosophy you are about to encounter.

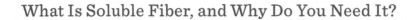

What Is Soluble Fiber, and Why Do You Need It?

Soluble fiber is known to slow things down in your digestive tract and is very good at absorbing things along the way. According to a 2010 paper published in *Nutrients*, these two characteristics are good for your heart because:

- Soluble fiber reduces the insulin response from a meal, which also reduces your liver's production of cholesterol.
- Soluble fiber attaches to fatty bile acids in your gastrointestinal tract, which your body must replace by using the cholesterol in your bloodstream.

Six Guidelines for Eating Heart Healthy

My goal here is to distill my heart-healthy eating philosophy into six primary messages that I'm confident will serve you in good stead for years to come.

1. **Lead with legumes.** According to a 2001 study published in the *Journal of the American Medical Association*, legume intake four times weekly is associated with a 22 percent reduction in heart-disease risk. I regularly tell my clients that I consider legumes to be one of the most underrated food groups for this very reason, owing largely to their high soluble fiber content, which is especially useful for keeping blood cholesterol levels down.

2. **Push the potassium.** High blood pressure is a major risk factor for heart disease and a leading cause of prescriptions in the United States. Whereas high dietary sodium levels may raise blood pressure, high dietary potassium levels, as discussed in a 2018 paper in *Hypertension*, can help restore

the balance. Potassium is found in high supply in commonly available foods such as bananas, tomatoes, potatoes, salmon, and avocado.

3. **Stick with soy.** A study published in the *European Journal of Preventive Cardiology* found soy intake to be associated with a reduced risk of heart disease and stroke, yet I know from my years of practice experience that not everyone loves soy-based foods. For those who do enjoy soy, there are some serious health benefits to be gained from the various protective compounds they contain, including polyphenols and isoflavones, both of which have strong antioxidant capabilities.

4. **Go nuts for tree nuts.** According to a 2017 paper in the *Journal of the American College of Cardiology*, regular tree nut intake reduces heart-disease risk by about 15 percent. Tree nuts are high in fiber, potassium, and different types of heart-healthy fats that are shown to improve cardiovascular health and reduce blood cholesterol and triglyceride levels. A 2020 paper published in the *Journal of the American Heart Association* recommends nut intake as an effective means of reducing heart-disease risk.

5. **Vegetables and fruits, fresh or frozen.** Fruits and vegetables are fundamental components of a heart-healthy diet. It won't be too surprising to hear that a 2017 paper in the *International Journal of Epidemiology* found that the consumption of these foods is strongly associated with a reduced risk of heart disease. I encourage you to enjoy both fresh and frozen fruits and vegetables. Eating fruits and vegetables of all varieties brings something to the table nutritionally. (Frozen mango is one of my favorites!)

6. **Get on omega-3s.** Omega-3 fatty acids are well known to have anti-inflammatory capabilities and also to lower blood triglyceride levels. A 2019 study published in the *Journal of the American Heart Association* showed that omega-3 intake did indeed reduce heart disease risk. The problem is that omega-3 fatty acids don't show up in too many foods. The primary contenders include flaxseed, chia seeds, walnuts, tofu, and commonly available fish such as salmon, trout, mackerel, and sardines.

Heart-Healthy Foods to Enjoy and Foods to Be Wary Of

In this section, I'd like to build and expand upon the heart-healthy tips that I provided by offering examples of the key foods I feel should play the largest role in your diet going forward, many of which will be strongly represented in the recipe section.

As you can probably tell by now, my nutrition philosophy is positively oriented, such that I prefer to spend our time telling you what to focus on, rather than what to avoid. With that being said, there are some key foods to be wary of on your heart-health journey, and I will point them out in this section as well.

Foods to Enjoy

Think of this section as a bit of a grocery list, not only because you will require these foods for many of the recipes in this book, but also because they represent the most important components of any heart-healthy diet, regardless of the way you choose to incorporate them. One might even say that you could eat these foods to your "heart's content."

Fruits high in soluble fiber. All types of berries, oranges, bananas, mangos, and kiwis are great examples of fruits that are high in soluble fiber. Fresh and frozen varieties are equally nutritious and can serve different purposes in your weekly routine.

Legumes, all types. Lentils, black beans, kidney beans, lima beans, white beans, chickpeas . . . all apply, and the list goes on. You can't go wrong with fresh or canned legumes; just be sure to look for "reduced-sodium" or "low-sodium" canned varieties and rinse them before use to reduce the salt content.

Olive and other oils. The question of which oil is best is always an interesting one when it comes to heart health. Among commonly available varieties, olive oil tends to be the highest in heart-healthy monounsaturated fats. Extra-virgin olive oil is great for cooking at low to medium heat (<350°F) or for dressing foods, whereas a light or refined olive oil is better for cooking at high heat (>375°F). Other oils that have a higher monounsaturated fat content and smoke point include avocado oil and peanut oil. According to a 2018 study published in *Open Heart*, the monounsaturated fats in these oils have a more beneficial effect on blood cholesterol and triglyceride levels than saturated fat–rich butter. Coconut oil, another popular oil, also contains saturated fats but from plant-based sources. A recent study published in the *British Medical Journal* found that the plant-based saturated fats in coconut oil, when compared with butter, are far better for cholesterol levels.

Omega-3–rich nuts/seeds. Only a few foods fit this bill, and they are flaxseed, chia seeds, and walnuts.

Other tree nuts/seeds. All other nut/seed varieties fit here, such as cashews, pistachios, Brazil nuts, chestnuts, almonds, sunflower seeds, pumpkin seeds, and so on. Be mindful of salted products. I'd recommend about ⅓ cup (50 grams) most days of the week.

Rolled oats. Although oatmeal in general is a heart-healthy food, owing to its high soluble fiber content, steel-cut oats take these benefits to the next level. They have a smaller effect on your blood sugar levels than instant varieties and may be a better choice for those living with prediabetes or type 2 diabetes. For those who don't like oatmeal, Kellogg's makes an excellent cholesterol-lowering cereal that is also great for blood sugar management: Kellogg's All-Bran Buds.

Sardines, salmon, mackerel, and trout. Most varieties of fish and seafood have some level of heart-healthy omega-3 fatty acids, but these four commonly available choices are near the top of the list. I'm a big fan of purchasing frozen fish for value and versatility.

Soy-based foods. Although soy-based foods are technically part of the legume family, I separate them here because they contain unique beneficial compounds that other legumes may not. The most commonly available soy-based foods include tofu, tempeh, soy milk, soybeans, and edamame.

Veggies high in soluble fiber. Include sweet potato, green beans, broccoli, Brussels sprouts, squash, collard greens, kale, and spinach in your heart-healthy diet. Once again, frozen varieties represent an economical and convenient alternative to fresh.

Foods to Be Wary Of

You can enjoy the following foods as part of a heart-healthy diet, but they may need to be moderated or modified if you turn to them on a regular basis.

Certain sauces, salad dressings, and condiments. From teriyaki sauce to ketchup and everything in between, these types of products tend to be high in sodium. The good news is that low-sodium varieties are available for many of them, and some can even be made at home. You'll find recipes for Tahini Dressing, Basil-Walnut Pesto, Marinara Sauce, Lemon Vinaigrette, and Yogurt-Herb Dressing in this book, all of which are used in other dishes throughout the book.

Pre-prepared high-sodium foods. Purchased frozen meals, soups, and pizzas tend to have very high sodium levels. The goal of this book is, of course, to get you to prepare stuff like this at home. You'll have plenty of easy recipes to help you do just that.

Processed red meat. Foods in this category include ham, hot dogs, sausages, corned beef, pepperoni, jerky, and related items. These foods should be limited because, compared with standard cuts of red meat, processed red meat products tend to be significantly higher in sodium, saturated fat, and harmful preservatives. A 2020 study published by *JAMA Internal Medicine* found that regular processed red meat consumption may increase heart disease risk by more than 40 percent.

Refined carbohydrates. Poor blood sugar control is a risk factor for heart disease. Items such as white rice, white bread, cornflakes, rice cakes, and various baked goods like pretzels and cookies tend to cause rapid increases in blood sugar levels. I appreciate that these foods do play cultural and sentimental roles for many people, so I don't expect you to exclude them flat-out. But I do encourage you to incorporate more whole grains in their place. Great examples include all-bran cereal, steel-cut oatmeal, brown rice, and whole-grain bread and bagels.

Flavor Hacks

I don't think you'll be surprised to hear this from a heart-health cookbook, but we are definitely aiming to moderate our use of sodium-rich seasonings, table salt included. It's not all bad news, though. There is a wide world of delicious herbs and spices at our disposal, many of which contain bioactive compounds that confer additional heart-health benefits.

These compounds, known as polyphenols, are strong antioxidants and, according to a 2013 paper published in *Nutrients*, are protective against cardiovascular disease. According to a paper published in *Current Atherosclerosis Reports*, polyphenols may have utility beyond their antioxidant function, such as relaxing the blood vessels and strengthening the immune system. Polyphenols are found in high amounts in some of the most flavorful herbs, spices, aromatics, and seasonings, including:

- Capers
- Cloves
- Garlic
- Lemon juice
- Onions
- Peppermint

- Rosemary
- Sage
- Shallot
- Thyme
- Vinegar

Many of the recipes in this book incorporate these items not only as salt-free flavor enhancers, but also as functional components of a heart-healthy diet.

The Easy, 5-Ingredient Promise

I know that time, money, and convenience are massive considerations when it comes to behavioral change. My commitment to 5-ingredient recipes is an acknowledgment of that fact, and I'm very confident the ease of preparation will really help simplify your transition to heart-healthier eating.

Please keep in mind that we do not count culinary essentials like salt, pepper, oil, or water in the 5-ingredient total. What you can expect to see, however, is a recipe collection that emphasizes the key foods discussed in the book thus far with an eye toward using familiar and easy-to-find items. This familiarity means less prep time, less grocery-shopping time, less cook time, and less stress, all of which will contribute to making your heart-healthy transition as painless as possible.

Even though the number of ingredients in any given recipe is limited, you'll see a wide variety of foods and flavors to ensure the dishes satisfy you for a long, long time.

Your Heart-Healthy Kitchen

My goal in this section is to briefly outline the key pieces of kitchen equipment that will be required for the majority of the recipes in the book and also to suggest a few other items that you don't necessarily need but would probably make your life easier.

Must-Have Equipment

You'll need the following items to prepare the recipes in this book.

- 8-inch square baking dish
- 9-by-13-inch baking dish
- Blender
- Chef's knife
- Colander
- Cutting board
- Pans
- Pots with lids
- Rimmed baking sheet
- Skewers
- Skillet (nonstick and/or oven-safe)
- Spatula
- Vegetable peeler
- Whisk
- Zester

Nice-to-Have Equipment

These items are not essential but are certainly nice to have.

- Food processor
- Grill
- Mandoline

- Pressure cooker
- Rice cooker
- Spiralizer

About the Recipes

I hope you've found the book equal parts entertaining and insightful so far. I've made a point of not giving you too many rules to follow, and I've homed in on some specific foods that are exceptionally good for the health of your heart. I've laid out some strong, specific guidance about nutrition and heart health, and the recipes to follow will bring this guidance to life in a manageable (and very tasty) way. As I've said, the book's 5-ingredient theme is honored throughout the recipe section, with extra emphasis placed on making your life as easy as possible as you delve into the world of heart-healthy eating.

My wonderful recipe developer, Katherine, and I have left no stone unturned in mapping out a delicious array of dishes that you can feel completely confident replicating in your own kitchen. Certain recipes will have special descriptive labels, including 30 minutes or less, one pot, vegan, or vegetarian. Many recipes will also be accompanied by tips that offer suggestions on preparing the recipe more quickly, modifying the ingredients to fit specific dietary restrictions, or even boosting or enhancing the flavor.

These tips and labels make the recipes more accessible to accommodate different tastes, needs, and time constraints because we fully appreciate that although heart health is the goal, each of us takes a slightly different path to get there.

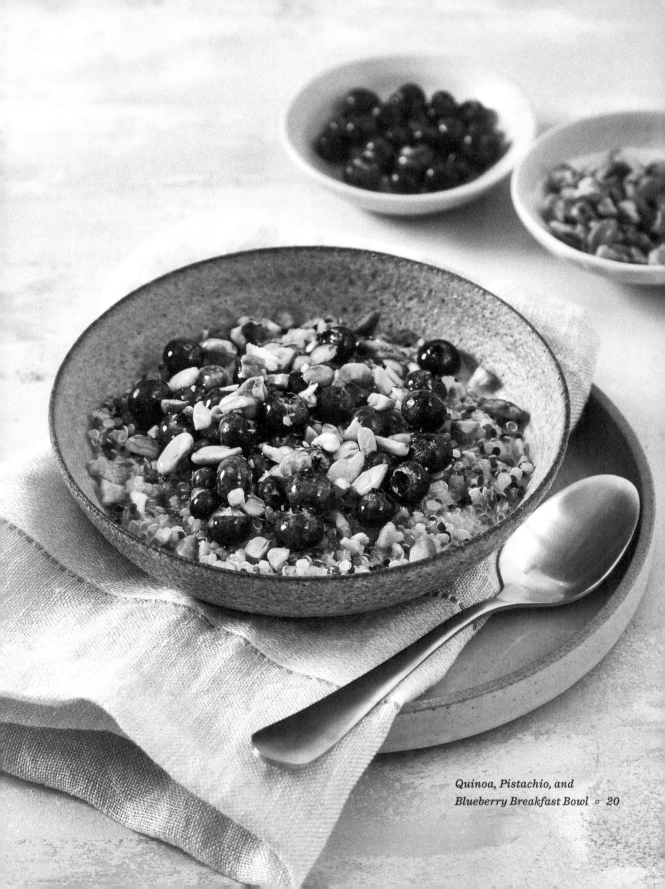

Quinoa, Pistachio, and
Blueberry Breakfast Bowl ○ 20

— CHAPTER TWO —

Breakfast and Beverages

Almond Butter and Blueberry Smoothie

30 MINUTES OR LESS ○ ONE POT ○ VEGAN ○ VEGETARIAN

Serves 2 / Prep time: 5 minutes

Heart-healthy almond butter is a great addition to your morning routine. A good source of vitamin E, magnesium, and riboflavin, almonds add a rich flavor and a creamy texture to this smoothie. If you have fresh berries, you can use them, too, but you will need to add a little more ice.

2 cups frozen blueberries

1¾ cups unsweetened
 almond milk

1 cup frozen spinach

¼ cup almond butter

½ cup ice

1. In a blender, combine the blueberries, almond milk, spinach, and almond butter. Process until smooth.

2. Add the ice, and blend again until smooth.

MAKE IT EASIER: Smoothies are quick to make, but if you want to cut out some of the prep in the morning, you can prepare individual resealable bags with blueberries and spinach and store them in the freezer. Just empty a bag into the blender in the morning along with the almond milk, almond butter, and ice when you're ready to make a smoothie.

Per Serving: Calories: 324; Total fat: 22g; Saturated fat: 1g; Sodium: 186mg; Carbohydrates: 29g; Fiber: 10g; Protein: 11g; Calcium: 671mg

Carrot, Ginger, and Kale Smoothie

30 MINUTES OR LESS ○ ONE POT ○ VEGAN ○ VEGETARIAN
Serves 2 / Prep time: 5 minutes

Smoothies are often loaded with sugars from fruit, but this veggie smoothie has a spicy savory appeal. Ginger is a powerful anti-inflammatory spice and a perfect addition to start your day. If you don't have a high-speed blender, grate the ginger on a zester or mince it before adding it to the blender.

2 cups chopped carrots

2 cups chopped kale

2 cups unsweetened
  almond milk

2 tablespoons
  ground flaxseed

1 (1½-inch) piece fresh
  ginger, peeled

½ cup ice

1. In a blender, combine the carrots, kale, almond milk, flaxseed, and ginger. Process for 1 to 2 minutes, or until smooth.

2. Add the ice, and blend again until smooth.

MAKE IT EASIER: Keep a bag of chopped carrots in the freezer to make the prep time for this smoothie even easier. Cut the amount of ice to just a couple cubes, and adjust with more as needed.

Per Serving: Calories: 139; Total fat: 8g; Saturated fat: 0g; Sodium: 210mg; Carbohydrates: 16g; Fiber: 7g; Protein: 5g; Calcium: 537mg

Overnight Oats with Walnuts and Berries

ONE POT ○ VEGAN ○ VEGETARIAN

Serves 4 / Prep time: 5 minutes + overnight to chill

Overnight oats are an easy way to ensure you get breakfast on busy mornings. Prepared in individual servings, these are ready to go when you need them. You can serve the oatmeal cold, or if you prefer a more traditional warmed oatmeal, simply heat the container in the microwave for about 1 minute, or until warmed through. Oats are packed with soluble fiber that helps lower LDL cholesterol, making them a heart-healthy start to your day.

1 cup rolled oats

1 cup unsweetened almond milk

2 tablespoons chia seeds

2 cups blueberries, blackberries, or chopped strawberries

½ cup chopped walnuts

1. Evenly distribute the oats, almond milk, and chia seeds into 4 small containers. Stir to mix well. Cover, and refrigerate overnight.

2. When ready to serve, top with ½ cup of berries and 2 tablespoons of walnuts each.

FLAVOR BOOST: Add a couple pinches ground cinnamon to the oats in step 1, or sweeten with 1 teaspoon of maple syrup or honey.

Per Serving: Calories: 338; Total fat: 16g; Saturated fat: 3g; Sodium: 60mg; Carbohydrates: 39g; Fiber: 9g; Protein: 11g; Calcium: 260mg

Cinnamon Chia Pudding with Berries

ONE POT ○ VEGAN ○ VEGETARIAN

Serves 4 / Prep time: 5 minutes + 2 hours to chill

Sweetened with honey, this simple breakfast pudding is filling and delicious. Use any seasonal berries or even other chopped fruits such as cherries, kiwi, mango, or peaches as toppings. For a little more protein, add a couple tablespoons of chopped nuts, like pistachios, cashews, almonds, or walnuts, on top. Chia seeds are high in protein, omega-3s, and fiber, which all contribute to heart health.

2 cups unsweetened almond milk

½ cup chia seeds

2 tablespoons honey

1 teaspoon ground cinnamon

Pinch salt

1 cup berries, such as blueberries, blackberries, raspberries, strawberries

1. In a medium bowl, whisk together the almond milk, chia seeds, honey, cinnamon, and salt to break up any clumps. Cover, and refrigerate for at least 2 hours, or until the pudding has thickened. Stir well.

2. Top with the berries.

MAKE IT EASIER: If you don't like the texture of chia seeds in the finished pudding, grind them up first to create a smooth pudding.

Per Serving: Calories: 207; Total fat: 11g; Saturated fat: 1g; Sodium: 139mg; Carbohydrates: 26g; Fiber: 11g; Protein: 5g; Calcium: 408mg

Muesli with Berries, Seeds, and Nuts

ONE POT ○ VEGAN ○ VEGETARIAN

Serves 4 / Prep time: 5 minutes / Cook time: 30 minutes

This simple dry cereal is easy to make and perfect for busy mornings. Served cold, the oat, sunflower seed, and almond mixture is crunchy and lightly browned in the oven and combines wonderfully with the natural sweetness of berries. Make a double batch, and enjoy it on busy mornings. Store the muesli in an airtight container for up to 1 month.

1 cup rolled oats

1 cup sunflower seeds

½ cup chopped almonds

Pinch salt

1 tablespoon extra-virgin olive oil

2 cups unsweetened almond milk

2 cups berries

1. Preheat the oven to 300°F. Line a baking sheet with parchment paper.

2. On the prepared baking sheet, combine the oats, sunflower seeds, almonds, and salt. Mix well.

3. Drizzle with the oil, and stir well. Spread the mixture in a thin layer.

4. Transfer the baking sheet to the oven, and bake, stirring once halfway through, for 30 minutes, or until the muesli is lightly browned. Remove from the oven. Set aside to cool.

5. Serve the muesli with the almond milk and berries.

FLAVOR BOOST: Stir 1 tablespoon of honey or maple syrup into the oats and nuts before baking to lightly sweeten the muesli.

Per Serving: Calories: 460; Total fat: 32g; Saturated fat: 3g; Sodium: 106mg; Carbohydrates: 34g; Fiber: 10g; Protein: 14g; Calcium: 303mg

Avocado and Tomato Toasts

30 MINUTES OR LESS ○ ONE POT ○ VEGETARIAN

Serves 2 / Prep time: 5 minutes / Cook time: 5 minutes

Avocado toast has been all the rage for years now, and with good reason. This simple and quick combination is loaded with heart-healthy monounsaturated fats and can help lower cholesterol. And when paired with the protein in the eggs and the sweetness of the tomato, it is also a delicious and filling meal that keeps you satisfied all morning.

1 tablespoon extra-virgin olive oil

2 large eggs

1 ripe avocado, pitted, peeled, and sliced

2 whole-wheat bread slices, toasted

Salt

Freshly ground black pepper

Pinch red pepper flakes

1 large tomato, thinly sliced

1. In a skillet, heat the oil over medium heat.

2. Carefully crack the eggs into the skillet, and fry for 3 to 4 minutes. Flip, and cook for 30 seconds, or until cooked to your desired doneness. Turn off the heat. Remove the eggs from the skillet.

3. Divide the avocado evenly between the pieces of toast. Using a fork, mash the avocado gently onto the bread. Season with salt, pepper, and a pinch of red pepper flakes.

4. Top with the tomato slices and eggs.

FLAVOR BOOST: Flavorful sprouts or microgreens are a nice addition here if you have them. Alternatively, some thinly sliced basil or cilantro leaves are a great topper on these toasts as well.

Per Serving: Calories: 411; Total fat: 28g; Saturated fat: 6g; Sodium: 302mg; Carbohydrates: 29g; Fiber: 12g; Protein: 14g; Calcium: 104mg

Quinoa, Pistachio, and Blueberry Breakfast Bowl

30 MINUTES OR LESS ∘ ONE POT ∘ VEGETARIAN

Serves 4 / Prep time: 5 minutes / Cook time: 20 minutes

Quinoa is easy to digest and is a complete protein, making it a great option for vegetarians. It is also quick cooking and easy to prepare, so it's perfect for mornings when you are short on time. This protein-packed breakfast bowl can be served warm or cold. There is no need to prepare the quinoa the morning of, since it reheats easily in the microwave and can be stored for up to 5 days in the refrigerator once cooked.

1¾ cups water

1 cup quinoa

Pinch salt

2 cups blueberries

½ cup shelled pistachios

1 cup unsweetened almond milk

4 teaspoons honey

1. In a saucepan, combine the water, quinoa, and salt. Bring to a boil.

2. Reduce the heat to a simmer. Cover the saucepan, and cook for 15 minutes, or until the water has been absorbed. Remove from the heat. Let sit for 5 minutes.

3. Evenly distribute the quinoa (about ¾ cup each), blueberries, and pistachios among 4 bowls.

4. Pour the almond milk on top, and drizzle with the honey.

SUBSTITUTION TIP: For a richer quinoa bowl, use ¼ cup of full-fat coconut milk in place of the almond milk.

Per Serving: Calories: 313; Total fat: 10g; Saturated fat: 1g; Sodium: 33mg; Carbohydrates: 48g; Fiber: 6g; Protein: 10g; Calcium: 141mg

Tofu "Egg" and Veggie Scramble

30 MINUTES OR LESS ◦ ONE POT ◦ VEGAN ◦ VEGETARIAN

Serves 4 / Prep time: 5 minutes / Cook time: 5 minutes

Tofu is a great egg substitute, and when paired with nutritional yeast, it has a nutty, cheesy flavor. Tofu is a good plant-based source of unsaturated fat and protein and is rich in isoflavones, which have been shown to lower the risk of heart disease. Serve this "egg" on its own, or scoop into a tortilla to make a breakfast wrap. Although many tofu recipes press the tofu before using to extract its moisture, in this recipe we cook the water out of the tofu in the pan, leaving the tofu coated in the spices and cooked perfectly.

1 tablespoon extra-virgin olive oil

1 (14-ounce) package firm tofu, drained

1 tablespoon nutritional yeast

½ teaspoon ground turmeric

½ teaspoon garlic powder

2 tablespoons chopped scallions (green and white parts), fresh chives, fresh cilantro, or fresh parsley

1. In a medium skillet, heat the oil over medium heat.

2. Crumble the tofu into the skillet, and cook for 2 minutes, or until heated through.

3. Add the nutritional yeast, turmeric, and garlic powder. Mix well. Continue to cook for 3 to 4 minutes, or until most of the water has cooked off the tofu. Remove from the heat.

4. Serve the scramble topped with the fresh herbs.

FLAVOR BOOST: Any number of additions can take this tofu to the next level. Spinach, kale, thinly sliced broccoli or cauliflower, or roasted vegetables from last night's dinner are all great for bulking up this scramble.

Per Serving: Calories: 132; Total fat: 9g; Saturated fat: 1g; Sodium: 142mg; Carbohydrates: 4g; Fiber: 1g; Protein: 11g; Calcium: 180mg

Eggs over Sautéed Tomato, Bell Pepper, and Zucchini

30 MINUTES OR LESS ○ ONE POT ○ VEGETARIAN

Serves 4 / Prep time: 10 minutes / Cook time: 15 minutes

Bell peppers are rich in vitamin C, beta-carotene, and vitamin K, making them a flavorful and nutritious addition to any dish. Combined with zucchini and tomato, this dish is a filling and quick veggie scramble that is reminiscent of ratatouille.

2 tablespoons extra-virgin olive oil, divided	1 medium zucchini, chopped	Salt
1 bell pepper, any color, cored and chopped	1 large tomato, chopped	Freshly ground black pepper
	½ teaspoon Italian seasoning	8 large eggs

1. In a large skillet, heat 1 tablespoon of oil over medium-high heat.

2. Add the bell pepper and zucchini. Cook for 3 to 4 minutes, or until starting to soften.

3. Add the tomato, and cook for 3 to 5 minutes, or until softened.

4. Add the Italian seasoning, and mix well. Season lightly with salt and pepper. Divide among 4 plates.

5. In the same skillet, heat the remaining 1 tablespoon of oil over medium heat.

6. Crack the eggs into the skillet, and fry for 3 to 4 minutes. Flip, and fry for 30 seconds, or to your preferred doneness. Remove from the heat.

7. Serve 2 eggs on top of each plate of cooked vegetables.

Per Serving: Calories: 232; Total fat: 17g; Saturated fat: 4g; Sodium: 188mg; Carbohydrates: 7g; Fiber: 2g; Protein: 14g; Calcium: 74mg

Omelet with Zucchini, Mushrooms, and Peppers

30 MINUTES OR LESS ◦ VEGETARIAN

Serves 2 / Prep time: 10 minutes / Cook time: 10 minutes

Omelets are a great vehicle for serving up a good dose of vegetables first thing in the morning. When making an omelet with crisp ingredients, it is important to cook the ingredients in advance. If time is an issue in the morning, you can make the filling the night before and add a minute more to the cooking time after folding the omelet to allow it to heat through.

1 tablespoon extra-virgin olive oil

½ small zucchini, chopped

1 cup sliced mushrooms

½ cup chopped cored bell pepper

1 teaspoon fresh thyme leaves

Salt

Freshly ground black pepper

4 large eggs

1. In a large nonstick skillet, heat the oil over medium heat.

2. Add the zucchini, mushrooms, and bell pepper. Sauté for 5 to 6 minutes, or until softened and lightly browned.

3. Stir in the thyme. Season lightly with salt and pepper. Transfer to a plate.

4. In a small bowl, whisk the eggs. Season lightly with salt and pepper.

5. Pour the eggs into the same skillet, and cook for 2 to 3 minutes over medium heat, or until set.

6. Place the vegetables on one side of the eggs, and fold the other side over them. Cook for about 1 minute, then using a spatula, flip to the other side to heat through. Remove from the heat. Divide the omelet evenly onto 2 plates, and serve.

Per Serving: Calories: 223; Total fat: 17g; Saturated fat: 4g; Sodium: 225mg; Carbohydrates: 4g; Fiber: 1g; Protein: 14g; Calcium: 64mg

Vegetable Frittata

30 MINUTES OR LESS ∘ VEGETARIAN

Serves 2 / Prep time: 10 minutes / Cook time: 20 minutes

A frittata is an open-faced omelet with the ingredients baked right in. Once you have the eggs in the pan, you can set a timer and clean up the kitchen while it finishes cooking in the oven. Asparagus is rich in bioflavonoids and glutathione, which are known to be strengthening to the immune system and have powerful antioxidant properties.

1 tablespoon extra-virgin olive oil

½ cup chopped asparagus

½ cup sliced zucchini

4 large eggs

Salt

Freshly ground black pepper

2 scallions, green and white parts, sliced

1 tablespoon chopped fresh dill

1. Preheat the oven to 375°F.

2. In a medium oven-safe skillet, heat the oil over medium-high heat.

3. Add the asparagus, and sauté for 2 to 3 minutes, or until nearly fork tender.

4. Add the zucchini, and cook for 2 to 3 minutes, or until tender.

5. In a small bowl, whisk the eggs. Season with salt and pepper. Pour over the vegetables in the skillet. Let the eggs set on the bottom for about 1 minute.

6. Sprinkle with the scallions and dill. Turn off the heat.

7. Transfer the skillet to the oven, and bake for 10 minutes, or until the eggs have cooked through and set. Remove from the oven. Cut the frittata in half.

Per Serving: Calories: 223; Total fat: 16g; Saturated fat: 4g; Sodium: 225mg; Carbohydrates: 5g; Fiber: 2g; Protein: 14g; Calcium: 83mg

Shakshuka

In shakshuka, a red sauce made of tomatoes and red bell peppers is used to poach eggs for a comforting meal to start your day. Seasoned with the warming flavor of cumin, this dish is best served with a piece of whole-grain crusty bread to sop up the juices. Tomatoes and red peppers are both rich in lycopene, which has been linked to a reduced risk of cardiovascular disease.

1 tablespoon extra-virgin olive oil

1 red bell pepper, chopped

1 (28-ounce) can low-sodium diced tomatoes

1 teaspoon ground cumin

Salt

Freshly ground black pepper

4 large eggs

¼ cup chopped fresh parsley

1. In a large skillet, heat the oil over medium-high heat.

2. Add the bell pepper, and cook for 4 to 6 minutes, or until softened.

3. Add the tomatoes with their juices and the cumin. Bring to a simmer. Cook for 10 minutes, or until the flavors meld and the sauce thickens. Season with salt and pepper.

4. Using a large spoon, make 4 depressions in the tomato mixture. Crack an egg into each depression. Cover the skillet, and cook for 5 to 7 minutes, depending on your desired doneness. Remove from the heat.

5. Serve the shakshuka topped with the parsley.

FLAVOR BOOST: Top the shakshuka with ½ cup of crumbled feta cheese.

Per Serving: Calories: 146; Total fat: 9g; Saturated fat: 2g; Sodium: 102mg; Carbohydrates: 10g; Fiber: 5g; Protein: 8g; Calcium: 106mg

Sweet Potato and Turkey Hash

Serves 4 / Prep time: 5 minutes / Cook time: 25 minutes

A simple seasoning of fennel turns low-fat ground turkey into a tasty sausage stand-in without all the added sodium in store-bought versions. Leave the skin on the sweet potatoes since it adds both fiber and a nice texture to the finished dish.

2½ tablespoons extra-virgin olive oil, divided

12 ounces ground turkey

½ teaspoon ground fennel seed

Salt

Freshly ground black pepper

1 pound sweet potato, diced

4 large eggs

¼ cup chopped fresh parsley

1. In a large skillet, heat 1 tablespoon of oil over medium-high heat.

2. Add the turkey, and cook, stirring regularly, for 4 to 6 minutes, or until cooked through.

3. Stir in the ground fennel. Season with salt and pepper. Transfer to a plate.

4. In the same skillet, heat 1 tablespoon of oil over medium-high heat.

5. Add the sweet potato, and cook for 10 to 12 minutes, or until cooked through and browned.

6. Return the turkey to the skillet, mix well, then divide the hash among 4 plates.

7. Pour the remaining ½ tablespoon of oil into the skillet, and heat over medium-high heat.

8. Crack the eggs into the skillet, and cook for 3 minutes, or until set.

9. Flip the eggs, and cook for 30 seconds to 1 minute, or to your desired doneness. Remove from the heat.

10. Top each portion with an egg, and garnish with the parsley.

MAKE IT EASIER: Look for chopped frozen sweet potatoes in the freezer section, and speed up prep time by eliminating the dicing.

Per Serving: Calories: 374; Total fat: 20g; Saturated fat: 5g; Sodium: 233mg; Carbohydrates: 24g; Fiber: 4g; Protein: 24g; Calcium: 88mg

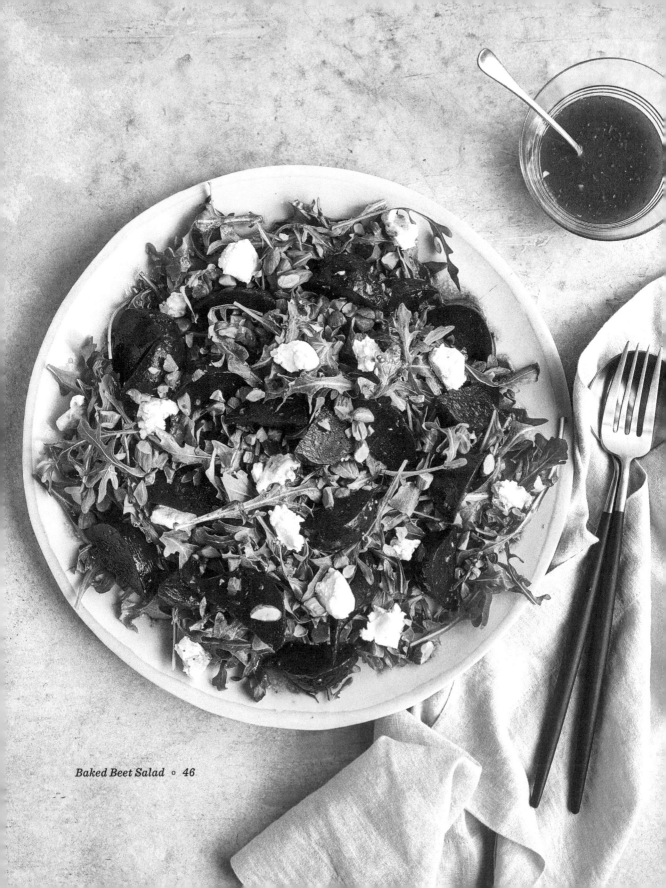

Baked Beet Salad ∘ 46

CHAPTER THREE

Snacks, Salads, and Sides

Roasted Lentil Snack Mix

VEGETARIAN

*Serves 4 / Prep time: 5 minutes + 1 hour 10 minutes to soak and dry /
Cook time: 25 minutes*

Lentils are packed with protein and fiber, both of which contribute to heart health, so any additional way to eat them is always a bonus. This snack mix is easy to make, nutritious, and affordable. Look for red lentils in the natural food section of your grocery store. They are a split lentil and are quicker cooking than other varieties. In this recipe, they need to be rehydrated by soaking in water.

1 cup dried red lentils

1 cup whole unsalted shelled pistachios

½ cup unsalted shelled sunflower seeds

½ cup dried cherries

½ cup dark chocolate chips

1. In a bowl, cover the lentils with water, and soak for 1 hour. Drain.

2. Preheat the oven to 350°F.

3. Transfer the lentils to a clean kitchen towel, and dab gently. Set aside for about 10 minutes to dry.

4. Spread the lentils out on a large baking sheet.

5. Transfer the baking sheet to the oven, and bake, stirring once or twice, for 20 to 25 minutes, or until the lentils are crisp. Remove from the oven. Let cool to room temperature. Transfer to a large bowl.

6. Add the pistachios, sunflower seeds, cherries, and chocolate chips. Toss to combine.

7. Let cool, and store in an airtight container at room temperature for up to 1 month.

SUBSTITUTION TIP: Use any type of dried fruit you like in place of the cherries. If you are using larger dried fruit that needs to be cut into smaller pieces, after cutting, toss in a teaspoon of rice flour to prevent sticking and clumping.

Per Serving: Calories: 629; Total fat: 32g; Saturated fat: 7g; Sodium: 12mg; Carbohydrates: 67g; Fiber: 13g; Protein: 23g; Calcium: 87mg

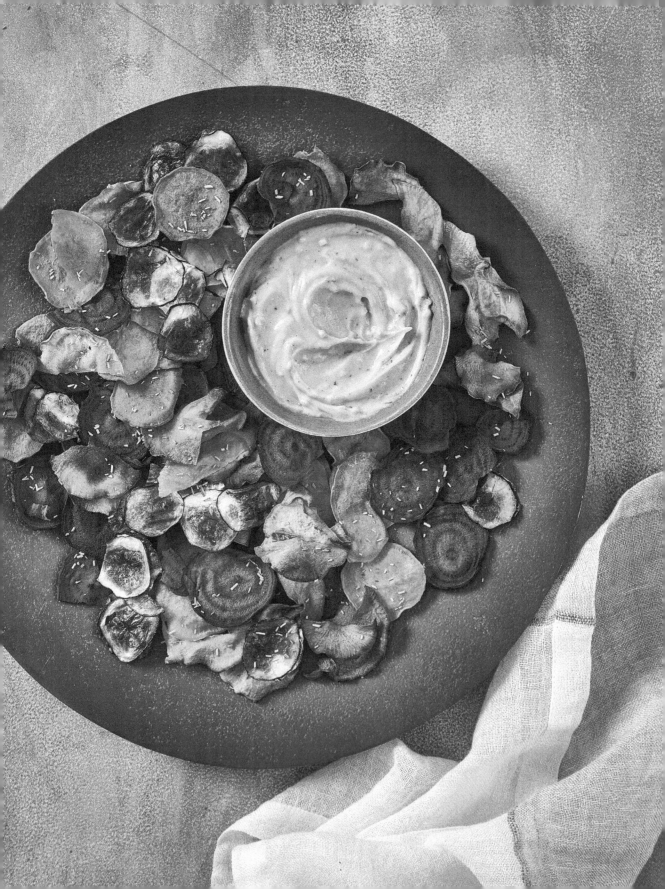

Vegetable Chips with Rosemary Salt

VEGAN ◦ VEGETARIAN

Serves 4 / Prep time: 15 minutes + 10 minutes to sit / Cook time: 50 minutes

Potato chips are a classic snack food that many people have a hard time giving up. Make these vegetable chips to transform the guilty pleasure into a healthy snack. A mandoline makes creating uniform slices simple, but if you don't have one, slice the vegetables as thinly and evenly as possible. Because of differences in size, you may need to cook the chips a little more or a little less; keep a close eye on them toward the end of the cooking time to ensure a browned, crisp chip.

Olive oil cooking spray

2 medium beets, peeled and sliced

1 medium zucchini, sliced

1 medium sweet potato, sliced

1 small rutabaga, peeled and sliced

½ teaspoon salt, plus more to sweat the vegetables

¼ teaspoon dried rosemary

1. Preheat the oven to 300°F. Spray a baking sheet with cooking spray. Line a plate with paper towels.

2. Lay the beets, zucchini, sweet potato, and rutabaga in a single layer on a paper towel. Lightly salt, and let sit for 10 minutes.

3. Cover the vegetables with another paper towel, and blot away any moisture on top.

4. Arrange the vegetables on the prepared baking sheet, and spray with cooking spray.

5. Transfer the baking sheet to the oven, and cook for 30 to 40 minutes, or until the vegetables have browned.

6. Flip the vegetables, and cook for 10 minutes, or until crisped. Remove from the oven. Transfer to the prepared plate to drain any excess oil.

continued

Vegetable Chips with Rosemary Salt *continued*

7. In a small bowl, mix together the salt and rosemary.

8. Lightly season the chips with the rosemary salt.

FLAVOR BOOST: Serve with Yogurt-Tahini Dip (page 149).

Per Serving: Calories: 72; Total fat: 0g; Saturated fat: 0g; Sodium: 350mg; Carbohydrates: 16g; Fiber: 4g; Protein: 2g; Calcium: 45mg

Roasted Chickpeas

ONE POT ○ VEGAN ○ VEGETARIAN

Serves 4 / Prep time: 5 minutes / Cook time: 30 minutes

This crunchy snack is just the thing to satisfy your midday hunger. Chickpeas are loaded with fiber, which helps reduce the cholesterol levels in blood and support heart health, making them perfect for snacking. Because they are so easy to make and don't keep especially well, make them as you need them for the best crunch, and once cooled, store them at room temperature in a loosely covered container for 1 to 2 days.

1 (15-ounce) can chickpeas, drained and rinsed

1 teaspoon extra-virgin olive oil

¼ teaspoon ground cumin

¼ teaspoon paprika

Salt

Freshly ground black pepper

1. Preheat the oven to 400°F. Line a baking sheet with parchment paper.

2. Using a clean kitchen towel, dry the chickpeas well. If any of the skins come off, discard them.

3. Transfer the chickpeas to the prepared baking sheet.

4. Add the oil, and toss.

5. Transfer the baking sheet to the oven, and roast for 25 to 30 minutes, or until the chickpeas are crisp and browned. Remove from the oven.

6. Add the cumin and paprika. Toss to combine. Season lightly with salt and pepper.

SUBSTITUTION TIP: The cumin and paprika can be replaced with any combination of different flavors based on what you like. Curry powder, onion and garlic powders, and nutritional yeast are all good on roasted chickpeas.

Per Serving: Calories: 89; Total fat: 3g; Saturated fat: 0g; Sodium: 160mg; Carbohydrates: 13g; Fiber: 4g; Protein: 4g; Calcium: 26mg

Homemade Nut Bars

VEGAN ○ VEGETARIAN

Makes 12 bars / Prep time: 5 minutes + 1 hour to cool / Cook time: 40 minutes

There are many varieties of energy, snack, and protein bars available at most stores, but you can also make these super easily at home and avoid all the additives. Using nuts, seeds, and maple syrup, these bars take just minutes to prep and will save you when hunger strikes. Store the leftover bars in an airtight container at room temperature for 1 week or in the refrigerator for up to 1 month.

1 cup chopped roasted unsalted almonds

½ cup roasted unsalted peanuts

½ cup puffed whole-grain cereal

¼ cup sesame seeds

Pinch salt

¼ cup maple syrup

1. Preheat the oven to 325°F. Line an 8-inch baking dish with parchment paper.

2. In a large bowl, combine the almonds, peanuts, cereal, sesame seeds, and salt. Toss to combine.

3. Stir in the maple syrup, and mix until well incorporated.

4. Transfer the mixture to the prepared baking dish. Using a spatula, press it down until tightly packed and the surface is even.

5. Transfer the baking dish to the oven, and bake for 40 minutes, or until the bars have lightly browned. Remove from the oven. Let cool at room temperature for 1 hour.

6. Lift the parchment paper out of the baking dish, and using a sharp knife, cut into 12 bars.

SUBSTITUTION TIP: To make this gluten-free, use a puffed cereal grain or any blend of grains that does not contain wheat, rye, or barley, such as millet or quinoa.

Per Serving: Calories: 432; Total fat: 33g; Saturated fat: 4g; Sodium: 48mg; Carbohydrates: 27g; Fiber: 7g; Protein: 14g; Calcium: 130mg

Simple Green Salad

30 MINUTES OR LESS ○ ONE POT ○ VEGAN ○ VEGETARIAN

Serves 4 / Prep time: 10 minutes

Romaine lettuce works well in this quick tossed salad, but any type of green leafy lettuce can be used here. Serve this dish as a side salad, or top it with grilled chicken or canned tuna to make it a light meal. If you are not serving this immediately, store the salad and the vinaigrette in separate containers until ready to serve, then toss right before serving.

1 head romaine or green
 leaf lettuce, chopped

1 large tomato, halved and
 thinly sliced

¼ cup sliced
 Kalamata olives

¼ cup sliced peperoncini

¼ cup Balsamic Vinaigrette
 (page 147)

1. In a large bowl, toss together the lettuce, tomato, olives, and peperoncini.

2. Drizzle the vinaigrette over the salad, and toss to combine. Serve immediately.

MAKE IT EASIER: If you want to skip the prep of chopping a head of lettuce, use 1 (8-ounce) bag of chopped romaine lettuce in place of the head of lettuce.

Per Serving: Calories: 122; Total fat: 10g; Saturated fat: 1g; Sodium: 142mg; Carbohydrates: 6g; Fiber: 2g; Protein: 2g; Calcium: 50mg

Sautéed Kale with Toasted Pine Nuts

30 MINUTES OR LESS ∘ ONE POT ∘ VEGAN ∘ VEGETARIAN

Serves 4 / Prep time: 10 minutes / Cook time: 15 minutes

Kale is a nutrient-dense leafy green that is rich in beta-carotene, vitamins A and C, and chlorophyll and has been studied for its cholesterol-lowering effects, which are enhanced when kale is cooked. Enjoy it regularly on your table in this simple sauté that takes just minutes to complete. The dark green, narrow dinosaur kale is my favorite variety, but curly or Russian kale can also be used in this dish.

¼ cup pine nuts

2 tablespoons extra-virgin olive oil

3 garlic cloves, minced

1 bunch kale, stemmed and chopped

Juice of 1 lemon

Salt

Freshly ground black pepper

1. Put the pine nuts in a large skillet, and toast over medium heat for 3 to 5 minutes, or until lightly browned. Remove from the skillet.

2. In the same skillet, heat the oil over medium-high heat.

3. Add the garlic, and sauté for 30 seconds, or until fragrant.

4. Add the kale, and cook, stirring regularly, for 5 to 7 minutes, or until tender. Season lightly with salt and pepper. Remove from the heat.

5. Sprinkle the pine nuts over the kale.

MAKE IT EASIER: To speed up prep, you can purchase a bag of prewashed cut kale or baby kale. If you use baby kale, cut the cook time to 3 to 5 minutes, or until the kale has just wilted.

Per Serving: Calories: 172; Total fat: 14g; Saturated fat: 1g; Sodium: 78mg; Carbohydrates: 12g; Fiber: 4g; Protein: 6g; Calcium: 157mg

Arugula Salad with Fennel

30 MINUTES OR LESS ○ ONE POT ○ VEGAN ○ VEGETARIAN

Serves 4 / Prep time: 10 minutes

Fennel is a bright and crunchy addition to a salad and pairs especially well with peppery arugula. If you need a quick salad to finish off your plate, this is a perfect go-to choice. Fennel and arugula both store well in the refrigerator for several days, so they are easy to keep on hand for quick salads. They are also both rich in fiber to help keep you fuller for longer and promote digestive health.

8 cups baby arugula

1 fennel bulb, cored and thinly sliced

3 tablespoons Lemon Vinaigrette (page 148)

¼ cup chopped hazelnuts

1. In a large bowl, toss together the arugula and fennel.

2. Drizzle with the vinaigrette, and toss again.

3. Serve the salad topped with the hazelnuts.

FLAVOR BOOST: Goat cheese pairs especially well with arugula. Add 1 or 2 tablespoons of crumbled goat cheese on top for a creamy burst of flavor.

Per Serving: Calories: 163; Total fat: 14g; Saturated fat: 1g; Sodium: 152mg; Carbohydrates: 8g; Fiber: 3g; Protein: 3g; Calcium: 103mg

Roasted Sweet Potato Fries

VEGAN ◦ VEGETARIAN

Serves 4 / Prep time: 10 minutes / Cook time: 35 minutes

Sweet potatoes are rich in fiber and antioxidants that support heart health, making them perfect for snacking, as a side dish, and as a healthier alternative to French fries. No need to peel the sweet potatoes since the skin adds fiber and also creates a crisp, tasty exterior.

2 large sweet potatoes, cut into thin fries

2 tablespoons extra-virgin olive oil

1 teaspoon garlic powder

½ teaspoon salt

Pinch ground cayenne pepper

1. Preheat the oven to 425°F. Line a baking sheet with parchment paper.

2. In a large bowl, toss together the sweet potatoes, oil, garlic powder, salt, and cayenne.

3. Spread the sweet potatoes out in an even layer on the prepared baking sheet.

4. Transfer the baking sheet to the oven, and bake, flipping once, for 30 to 35 minutes, or until the sweet potatoes are crisp. Remove from the oven.

FLAVOR BOOST: Serve the fries with Yogurt-Tahini Dip (page 149).

Per Serving: Calories: 123; Total fat: 7g; Saturated fat: 1g; Sodium: 328mg; Carbohydrates: 15g; Fiber: 2g; Protein: 1g; Calcium: 22mg

Roasted Peppers and Zucchini

ONE POT ○ VEGAN ○ VEGETARIAN

Serves 4 / Prep time: 10 minutes / Cook time: 30 minutes

Bell pepper and zucchini are both low-carb vegetables and a perfect pairing for a number of meat and vegetable dishes. Bell peppers are rich in vitamin B_6 and folic acid, which both help reduce the risk of heart disease. Italian seasoning—a simple blend of oregano, basil, thyme, rosemary, garlic powder, and sage—amps up the flavor.

2 small zucchini, sliced

2 bell peppers, cored and cut into 1-inch pieces

1 red onion, cut into 1-inch pieces

2 tablespoons extra-virgin olive oil

1 tablespoon freshly squeezed lemon juice

1 teaspoon Italian seasoning

Salt

Freshly ground black pepper

1. Preheat the oven to 425°F.

2. On a baking sheet, combine the zucchini, bell peppers, and onion.

3. Drizzle with the oil, lemon juice, and Italian seasoning. Toss to coat. Season with salt and pepper. Stir to combine.

4. Spread the vegetables in an even layer.

5. Transfer the baking sheet to the oven, and roast, tossing once about halfway through, for 30 minutes, or until the vegetables are tender and browned on the edges. Remove from the oven. Serve warm.

SUBSTITUTION TIP: Substitute 1 yellow summer squash for 1 zucchini for a little more color in the dish, and use 1 green and 1 red bell pepper for even more.

Per Serving: Calories: 107; Total fat: 7g; Saturated fat: 1g; Sodium: 47mg; Carbohydrates: 11g; Fiber: 2g; Protein: 2g; Calcium: 26mg

Polenta Cakes

VEGAN ○ VEGETARIAN

Serves 4 / Prep time: 5 minutes + 2 hours to chill / Cook time: 40 minutes

Polenta, or boiled cornmeal, originated in northern and central Italy and remains a staple of the cuisine today. Served either soft or cooked down and cooled until solid and then fried, as in this recipe, polenta is a versatile side dish that is a perfect vessel for sauces. Polenta is high in carbohydrates, so portion control is important; however, it's rich in fiber, making it a heart-healthy choice when served in moderation and prepared with olive oil instead of milk, cream, or cheese.

5 cups water

1 cup fine cornmeal

1 teaspoon garlic powder

¼ teaspoon salt

Olive oil cooking spray

2 tablespoons extra-virgin olive oil, divided

1. In a large saucepan, bring the water to a rolling boil over high heat.

2. While whisking, slowly pour the cornmeal into the water, and continue whisking until well combined.

3. Whisk in the garlic powder and salt.

4. Reduce the heat to a simmer. Cook, stirring regularly, for 25 to 30 minutes, or until the cornmeal has thickened. Remove from the heat.

5. Meanwhile, spray a 9-by-13-inch baking dish with cooking spray. Line with parchment paper.

6. Pour the mixture into the prepared dish. Using a spoon, smooth the surface. Refrigerate for at least 2 hours, or until solid.

7. Lift the parchment paper from the dish. Cut the polenta into 12 pieces, or use a cookie cutter to create circular cakes if desired.

8. In a large skillet, heat the oil over medium-high heat.

9. Working in batches, add the polenta cakes, and cook for 2 to 3 minutes per side, or until browned. Remove from the heat.

FLAVOR BOOST: You can add any number of seasonings to the polenta to amp up the flavor. Shredded Parmesan cheese or nutritional yeast and dried seasonings like onion powder, cayenne, oregano, basil, or thyme are all good additions.

Per Serving: Calories: 173; Total fat: 8g; Saturated fat: 1g; Sodium: 157mg; Carbohydrates: 24g; Fiber: 2g; Protein: 3g; Calcium: 3mg

Israeli Couscous Salad

30 MINUTES OR LESS ◦ VEGAN ◦ VEGETARIAN

Serves 6 / Prep time: 10 minutes / Cook time: 15 minutes

Israeli couscous, also called pearl couscous, is larger and chewier than the smaller quick-cooking couscous. Both are a type of dried pasta, but the larger pearl type benefits greatly from toasting lightly before cooking to really draw out a nutty flavor. Couscous is rich in selenium, which is an important mineral that helps decrease inflammation and repair damaged cells.

3 tablespoons extra-virgin olive oil, divided

2 tablespoons red-wine vinegar

½ teaspoon salt, divided

¼ teaspoon freshly ground black pepper

1 cup Israeli couscous

1 cup water

2 cups halved cherry tomatoes

1 (15-ounce) can chickpeas, drained and rinsed

¼ cup chopped fresh parsley

1. To make the vinaigrette, in a small bowl, whisk together 2 tablespoons of oil, the vinegar, ¼ teaspoon of salt, and the pepper.

2. In a large saucepan, heat the remaining 1 tablespoon of oil over medium-high heat.

3. Add the couscous, and cook, stirring, for 2 minutes, or until lightly browned.

4. Add the water. Bring to a boil.

5. Stir in the remaining ¼ teaspoon of salt.

6. Reduce the heat to a simmer. Cook for about 10 minutes, or until the couscous is tender. Remove from the heat. Drain, and set aside to cool.

7. In a large bowl, combine the tomatoes, chickpeas, and vinaigrette. Stir to combine.

8. Add the couscous, and mix again. Let cool to room temperature.

9. Stir in the parsley.

FLAVOR BOOST: If you eat dairy, feta cheese goes well with this salad. Sprinkle about 2 tablespoons of crumbled feta over each serving.

Per Serving: Calories: 231; Total fat: 8g; Saturated fat: 1g; Sodium: 282mg; Carbohydrates: 33g; Fiber: 5g; Protein: 7g; Calcium: 32mg

Baked Beet Salad

Serves 4 / Prep time: 10 minutes / Cook time: 35 minutes

Goat cheese and beets are tied together with a balsamic vinaigrette in this simple and naturally sweet salad. To deepen the flavor of the almonds, toast them in the oven for 5 to 7 minutes, or until lightly browned, while the beets bake. Arugula is a peppery green that pairs well with beets, but you can use any other salad greens you have on hand if needed. Beets are rich in betaine, a powerful compound that supports cardio health by lowering the concentration of homocysteine, which is harmful to blood vessels.

1 bunch (3 or 4 medium) beets

1 (8-ounce) bag arugula

¼ cup Balsamic Vinaigrette (page 147)

¼ cup chopped almonds

¼ cup crumbled goat cheese

1. Preheat the oven to 350°F.

2. Wash the beets well. Wrap them in aluminum foil.

3. Transfer the beets to the oven, and bake for 25 to 35 minutes, depending on the size of the beets, or until easily pierced with a fork. Remove from the oven. Let cool until easy to handle.

4. Using your hands, slide the skins off the beets, and discard. Cut the beets into wedges.

5. Put the beets in a large bowl with the arugula.

6. Drizzle the vinaigrette over the beets, and toss gently.

7. Serve the salad topped with the almonds and cheese.

MAKE IT EASIER: Beets can take a while to roast depending on their size, but you can speed things up by steaming them in a pressure cooker. Place 1 cup of water and the beets in the pressure cooker, and cook on manual for 15 minutes. When cooking is complete, quick-release the pressure.

Per Serving: Calories: 197; Total fat: 14g; Saturated fat: 2g; Sodium: 171mg; Carbohydrates: 16g; Fiber: 4g; Protein: 6g; Calcium: 137mg

Zucchini Noodles

30 MINUTES OR LESS ◦ ONE POT

Serves 4 / Prep time: 10 minutes / Cook time: 5 minutes

Zucchini noodles, or zoodles, are used as a low-carb alternative to pasta because of their ability to maintain their shape after a quick cooking. Zucchini is rich in vitamins A and C, folate, and fiber, making these simple zoodles a heart-healthy alternative to gluten-containing noodles. If you don't have a spiralizer, you can use a vegetable peeler to cut the zucchini into flat zoodles or cut them by hand into matchstick-size pieces for a similar effect.

2 tablespoons extra-virgin olive oil

2 garlic cloves, minced

2 medium zucchini, spiralized

½ teaspoon salt

½ teaspoon freshly ground black pepper

½ cup chopped fresh parsley

¼ cup shredded Parmesan cheese

1. In a large skillet, heat the oil over medium-high heat.

2. Add the garlic, and cook for about 30 seconds, or until fragrant.

3. Add the zucchini, salt, and pepper. Cook for 2 to 3 minutes, or until the noodles are just barely al dente. Remove from the heat.

4. Serve the noodles topped with the parsley and cheese.

SUBSTITUTION TIP: Butternut squash noodles are a good substitute for zucchini noodles and can be found in the prepared produce section of many grocery stores. Butternut squash takes a little longer to cook; sauté butternut squash noodles for 7 to 10 minutes, or until tender.

Per Serving: Calories: 108; Total fat: 9g; Saturated fat: 2g; Sodium: 416mg; Carbohydrates: 5g; Fiber: 1g; Protein: 3g; Calcium: 82mg

Lemon Rice

ONE POT ○ VEGAN ○ VEGETARIAN

Serves 4 / Prep time: 5 minutes + 10 minutes to rest / Cook time: 45 minutes

This is a flavorful way to turn ordinary brown rice into something special while still making it versatile enough to serve with just about any main dish. Lemon juice and zest brighten this dish with little effort, and aromatic dill adds a touch of color and flavor to the rice. Serve this instead of white rice for a whole-grain twist on the ordinary.

2 tablespoons extra-virgin olive oil

1 medium onion, chopped

2 cups low-sodium vegetable broth

1 cup brown rice

¼ cup freshly squeezed lemon juice

Zest of 1 lemon

½ teaspoon dried dill

1. In a large saucepan, heat the oil over medium-high heat.

2. Add the onion, and cook for 3 to 5 minutes, or until softened.

3. Add the broth, rice, and lemon juice. Bring to a boil.

4. Reduce the heat to a simmer. Cover the saucepan, and cook for 30 to 40 minutes, or according to the package directions and until the liquid has evaporated. Remove from the heat. Let rest, covered, for 10 minutes.

5. Stir in the lemon zest and dill.

MAKE IT EASIER: If you have a pressure cooker, cook the rice with the onion, broth, and lemon juice on high pressure for 15 minutes. When the cooking is complete, let the pressure release naturally for 5 minutes, then quick-release the remaining pressure, and continue with the recipe at step 5.

Per Serving: Calories: 246; Total fat: 8g; Saturated fat: 1g; Sodium: 3mg; Carbohydrates: 40g; Fiber: 2g; Protein: 4g; Calcium: 23mg

Quinoa Tabbouleh

VEGAN ○ VEGETARIAN

Serves 4 / Prep time: 10 minutes + 1 hour to chill / Cook time: 15 minutes

Tabbouleh is a classic grain salad traditionally made with bulgur, a type of cracked wheat. In this version, it gets a protein boost and is made gluten-free by substituting the bulgur with quinoa. Serve it as a side, or scoop a serving into a pita and top with Baba Ghanoush (page 142) or Garlic Hummus (page 141) for a complete vegan meal.

2 cups water	1 English cucumber, finely chopped	½ cup Lemon Vinaigrette (page 148)
1 cup quinoa		
¼ teaspoon salt	2 cups halved tomatoes	½ cup chopped fresh parsley

1. In a large saucepan, combine the water, quinoa, and salt. Bring to a boil.

2. Reduce the heat to simmer. Cover the saucepan, and cook for 10 minutes, or until the liquid has been absorbed and the quinoa is tender. Remove from the heat. Let rest, covered, for 5 minutes, then fluff with a fork.

3. In a large bowl, combine the cucumber, tomatoes, and vinaigrette. Toss well. Let sit until the quinoa is ready.

4. Add the quinoa, and toss well to combine.

5. Add the parsley, and toss again.

6. Refrigerate for 1 hour before serving. Toss to incorporate the vinaigrette again before serving.

FLAVOR BOOST: Add a can of drained and rinsed chickpeas to the tabbouleh to make this a more filling meal.

Per Serving: Calories: 356; Total fat: 21g; Saturated fat: 2g; Sodium: 375mg; Carbohydrates: 36g; Fiber: 5g; Protein: 7g; Calcium: 56mg

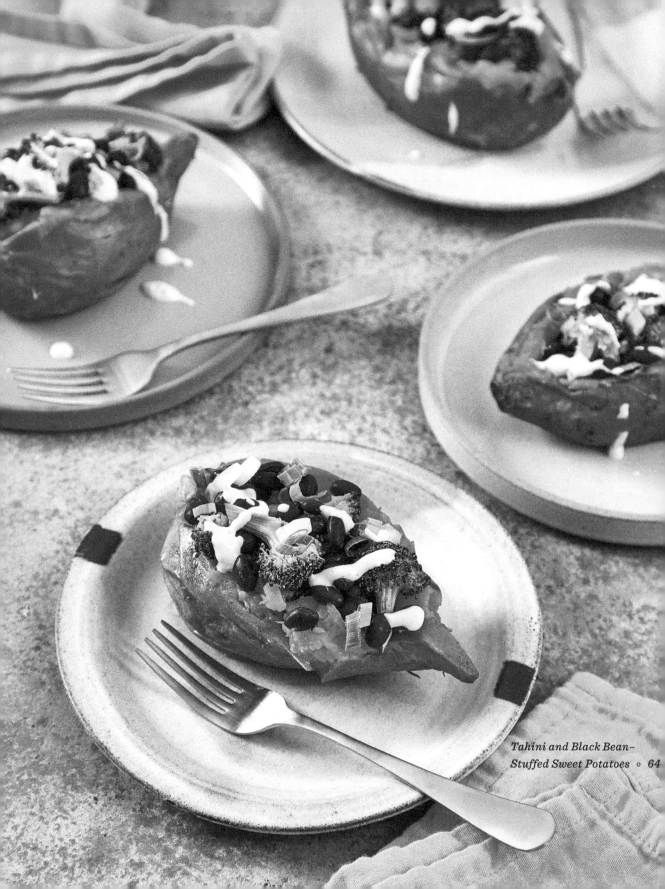

Tahini and Black Bean–
Stuffed Sweet Potatoes ∘ 64

Vegetarian and Vegan Mains

continued

Vegetarian and Vegan Mains

continued

Creamy Pumpkin Soup

30 MINUTES OR LESS ◦ VEGAN ◦ VEGETARIAN

Serves 4 / Prep time: 5 minutes / Cook time: 10 minutes

Pumpkin puree is a versatile ingredient that is rich in vitamins A and C and tastes great in soups and stews. Make sure to purchase pure pumpkin puree and not pumpkin pie filling, which has added sugar and spices. Tofu provides plant-based protein in this soup to help keep you fuller for longer and create the creamy texture.

3 cups vegetable broth, divided

7 ounces soft tofu

1 (15-ounce) can pumpkin puree

1 tablespoon grated fresh ginger

½ teaspoon ground cinnamon

Salt

Freshly ground black pepper

1. In a blender, combine 1 cup of broth and the tofu. Process until smooth.

2. In a large saucepan, combine the tofu, remaining 2 cups of broth, the pumpkin puree, ginger, and cinnamon. Bring to a boil.

3. Reduce the heat to a simmer. Cook for 10 minutes, or until the flavors meld. Remove from the heat. Season with salt and pepper.

FLAVOR BOOST: Add ¼ teaspoon of ground nutmeg and a pinch cayenne pepper for a deeper warming flavor.

Per Serving: Calories: 68; Total fat: 2g; Saturated fat: 0g; Sodium: 48mg; Carbohydrates: 10g; Fiber: 3g; Protein: 4g; Calcium: 86mg

Minestrone

30 MINUTES OR LESS ◦ ONE POT ◦ VEGAN ◦ VEGETARIAN

Serves 6 / Prep time: 10 minutes / Cook time: 20 minutes

This homestyle soup is often loaded with sodium when prepared in a restaurant, but this simple and quick version lets you adjust the soup to your taste. Kidney beans are an inexpensive plant-based protein that can aid in weight management and lower LDL cholesterol, making them a great base for soup. If you like, add a cup of cooked mini-shell pasta to the soup at the end of cooking.

6 cups Vegetable Stock (page 150) or store-bought low-sodium vegetable broth

2 (15-ounce) cans low-sodium kidney beans, drained and rinsed

1 (15-ounce) can diced tomatoes with Italian seasoning

1 cup finely chopped carrots

1 cup finely chopped celery

Salt

Freshly ground black pepper

In a large saucepan, combine the stock, beans, tomatoes with their juices, carrots, and celery. Bring to a simmer over medium heat. Cook for 15 minutes, or until the flavors meld. Remove from the heat. Season with salt and pepper.

FLAVOR BOOST: Sprinkle 1 or 2 tablespoons of shredded Parmesan cheese over the soup to serve.

Per Serving: Calories: 238; Total fat: 1g; Saturated fat: 0g; Sodium: 135mg; Carbohydrates: 44g; Fiber: 13g; Protein: 15g; Calcium: 96mg

Lentil and Veggie Soup

ONE POT ○ VEGAN ○ VEGETARIAN

Serves 4 / Prep time: 10 minutes / Cook time: 40 minutes

Lentils are quick cooking for a legume or bean, and they don't require soaking, making them a perfect solution for a weeknight meal. Lentils are high in folate, fiber, potassium, and polyphenols and have been studied extensively for their effects on lowering cholesterol, blood pressure, and blood glucose. This nourishing soup is simple to make from dried lentils, but if you prefer, you could also use 2 (15-ounce) cans, added in step 3, and reduce the cooking time in step 4 to about 10 minutes, or until the onion and carrots are tender.

2 tablespoons extra-virgin olive oil

1 medium onion, chopped

2 carrots, chopped

1 cup dried brown lentils

1 (28-ounce) can low-sodium diced tomatoes

4 cups water

Juice of 1 lemon

Salt

Freshly ground black pepper

1. In a large saucepan, heat the oil over medium-high heat.

2. Add the onion and carrots. Sauté for 3 to 5 minutes, or until just starting to soften.

3. Add the lentils, tomatoes with their juices, and water. Bring to a boil.

4. Reduce the heat to a simmer. Cook for 25 to 30 minutes, or until the lentils are tender. Remove from the heat.

5. Using an immersion blender, puree some of the soup, or remove 2 cups from the saucepan, process it in a blender, and return it to the saucepan.

6. Add the lemon juice. Season with salt and pepper.

Per Serving: Calories: 287; Total fat: 8g; Saturated fat: 1g; Sodium: 90mg; Carbohydrates: 44g; Fiber: 10g; Protein: 14g; Calcium: 99mg

White Bean Soup with Orange and Celery

30 MINUTES OR LESS ◦ ONE POT ◦ VEGAN ◦ VEGETARIAN

Serves 6 / Prep time: 10 minutes / Cook time: 25 minutes

This soup is flavored by an orange and its zest, which transforms this simple bean soup into something noteworthy. Celery is generously used in the soup, providing texture and flavor. Celery is anti-inflammatory, helps lower blood pressure, and is a good source of fiber, making it a perfect heart-healthy ingredient to feature in soup. But it is also one of the vegetables most highly contaminated with pesticides, so choose organic whenever possible.

2 tablespoons extra-virgin olive oil, plus more for serving

1 large onion, chopped

1½ cups chopped celery

½ teaspoon salt

½ teaspoon freshly ground black pepper

4 cups water

2 (15-ounce) cans white beans, drained and rinsed

1 teaspoon dried oregano

Zest of ½ medium orange

Juice of 1 medium orange

1. In a large saucepan, heat the oil over medium-high heat.

2. Add the onion and celery. Cook for 4 to 6 minutes, or until lightly browned and softened. Season with the salt and pepper.

3. Add the water, beans, and oregano. Bring to a boil.

4. Reduce the heat to a simmer. Cook for 15 minutes, or until the flavors meld. Remove from the heat.

5. Add the orange zest and orange juice.

6. Serve the soup topped with more oil if desired.

SUBSTITUTION TIP: This soup can also be made using the juice and zest from 1 lemon in place of the orange juice.

Per Serving: Calories: 188; Total fat: 5g; Saturated fat: 1g; Sodium: 217mg; Carbohydrates: 28g; Fiber: 10g; Protein: 9g; Calcium: 86mg

Smashed Chickpea Salad Sandwich

30 MINUTES OR LESS ◦ ONE POT ◦ VEGETARIAN

Serves 4 / Prep time: 10 minutes

This simple sandwich is reminiscent of a classic egg salad sandwich, but chickpeas replace the eggs for a protein-packed veggie sandwich like the original. Chickpeas are rich in a plant sterol named sitosterol that interferes with the body's cholesterol absorption, which helps lower overall cholesterol levels. If you want to make this recipe vegan, use coconut yogurt in place of the Greek yogurt.

1 (15-ounce) can low-sodium chickpeas, drained and rinsed

¼ cup finely chopped red onion

¼ cup plain, unsweetened, low-fat Greek yogurt

1½ teaspoons whole-grain mustard

Salt

Freshly ground black pepper

4 whole-grain bread slices

1. In a bowl, using a fork, mash the chickpeas coarsely, leaving some whole for texture.

2. Add the onion, yogurt, and mustard. Season with salt and pepper.

3. Divide the salad between 2 pieces of bread. Top with the remaining slices of bread.

FLAVOR BOOST: Add ½ teaspoon of turmeric to mimic the color of egg salad. Add lettuce or sprouts and sliced tomato to the sandwich to serve.

Per Serving: Calories: 162; Total fat: 3g; Saturated fat: 1g; Sodium: 287mg; Carbohydrates: 26g; Fiber: 6g; Protein: 8g; Calcium: 73mg

Lentil and Fennel Salad

30 MINUTES OR LESS ○ VEGAN ○ VEGETARIAN

Serves 4 / Prep time: 10 minutes / Cook time: 20 minutes

The licorice flavor of fennel and the sweetness of carrots combine well with the lentils here for a main course salad. Because the salad is composed largely of lentils, it is hearty and easy to make. When eating fennel fresh, as in this recipe, remove the outer layer of the fennel bulb before slicing the rest of the bulb very thinly.

1 cup dried brown or green lentils

2 carrots, grated

1 fennel bulb, cored and thinly sliced

½ cup chopped fresh parsley

½ cup Lemon Vinaigrette (page 148)

1. In a large saucepan, cover the lentils with water by a few inches. Bring to a boil over high heat.

2. Reduce the heat to medium. Simmer for 15 to 20 minutes, or until the lentils are tender but not mushy. Remove from the heat. Drain, and rinse with cold water to cool.

3. While the lentils are cooking, in a large bowl, toss together the carrots, fennel, parsley, and vinaigrette. Let sit until the lentils are ready.

4. Add the lentils, and gently mix.

SUBSTITUTION TIP: Celery can be used in place of the fennel for a similar effect. Be sure to slice it thinly if using.

Per Serving: Calories: 372; Total fat: 19g; Saturated fat: 2g; Sodium: 284mg; Carbohydrates: 41g; Fiber: 8g; Protein: 13g; Calcium: 72mg

White Bean Salad on Toast

30 MINUTES OR LESS ○ ONE POT ○ VEGAN ○ VEGETARIAN

Serves 4 / Prep time: 10 minutes

Simple salads are perfect for busy and hot days when you don't want to spend time over a stove and heat up the house. This version combines the crunch of cucumber with a flavorful lemon vinaigrette for a quick main course salad served over bread. It can be made in just about the time it takes to toast the bread.

1 (15-ounce) can low-sodium white beans, drained and rinsed

½ English cucumber, finely chopped

½ cup chopped tomatoes

½ cup Lemon Vinaigrette (page 148)

4 whole-grain thick crusty bread slices, toasted

Salt

Freshly ground black pepper

1. In a large bowl, toss together the beans, cucumber, and tomatoes.

2. Drizzle with the vinaigrette, and mix well.

3. Divide the salad on top of the bread slices. Season lightly with salt and pepper.

FLAVOR BOOST: Peel a large garlic clove, and rub it over each piece of toast to add a spicy garlic flavor to the dish. Sprinkle the finished toasts with 2 tablespoons of chopped fresh herbs, such as parsley or cilantro.

Per Serving: Calories: 363; Total fat: 20g; Saturated fat: 2g; Sodium: 525mg; Carbohydrates: 37g; Fiber: 7g; Protein: 11g; Calcium: 93mg

Artichoke Heart and Chickpea–Stuffed Portabellas

VEGAN ○ VEGETARIAN

Serves 4 / Prep time: 10 minutes / Cook time: 30 minutes

Artichoke hearts are a good source of fiber and bring a lot of distinctive flavor to this dish. Portabella mushrooms are the perfect size for stuffing, making this an easy meal. We're not using the mushroom stems, but that doesn't mean you need to throw them away. Chop them up and use them in stir-fry dishes, or mix them into your breakfast scramble for an extra boost of vitamin D.

4 large portabella mushrooms, stemmed

1 tablespoon extra-virgin olive oil

1 (15-ounce) can low-sodium chickpeas, drained and rinsed

1 cup cooked brown rice or Lemon Rice (page 49)

½ red bell pepper, cored and finely chopped

½ cup chopped artichoke hearts

Salt

Freshly ground black pepper

1. Preheat the oven to 350°F.

2. Place the mushrooms, gill-side down, on a large baking sheet.

3. Drizzle with the oil.

4. Transfer the baking sheet to the oven, and bake for 10 minutes. Flip the mushrooms, and bake for 10 minutes, or until tender. Remove from the oven, leaving the oven on.

5. In a large bowl, combine the chickpeas, rice, bell pepper, and artichoke hearts. Season with salt and pepper.

6. Divide the mixture among the mushrooms.

7. Return the baking sheet to the oven, and bake for 10 more minutes, or until the filling is heated through. Remove from the oven.

SUBSTITUTION TIP: Half a cup of oil-packed sun-dried tomatoes can be used in place of the red bell pepper.

Per Serving: Calories: 194; Total fat: 6g; Saturated fat: 1g; Sodium: 181mg; Carbohydrates: 29g; Fiber: 7g; Protein: 8g; Calcium: 47mg

Tahini and Black Bean–
Stuffed Sweet Potatoes

VEGAN ○ VEGETARIAN

Serves 4 / Prep time: 10 minutes / Cook time: 30 minutes

The tahini dressing really sets off this flavor combination with its rich creamy garlic flavor, and with a combination of beans, sweet potato, and broccoli, this is one nutrient-dense plant-based meal. This dish keeps well in the refrigerator, so you can prep a batch of these sweet potatoes and enjoy them throughout the week for easy lunches.

4 medium sweet potatoes

1 tablespoon extra-virgin olive oil, divided

2 cups broccoli florets

Salt

Freshly ground black pepper

1 (15-ounce) can low-sodium black beans, drained and rinsed

½ cup Tahini Dressing (page 145)

2 scallions, green and white parts, sliced

1. Preheat the oven to 375°F.

2. Using a fork, prick the sweet potatoes 2 or 3 times.

3. Rub the skin with ½ tablespoon of oil.

4. Put the sweet potatoes on a baking sheet.

5. Transfer the baking sheet to the oven, and bake for 20 to 30 minutes, depending on their size, or until the sweet potatoes are easily pierced using a fork.

6. Meanwhile, in a medium bowl, toss together the broccoli and remaining ½ tablespoon of oil. Season lightly with salt and pepper.

7. After the sweet potatoes have been cooking for about 10 minutes, add the broccoli to the baking sheet alongside the sweet potatoes, and roast for 20 minutes, or until the broccoli is tender and browned. Remove the baking sheet from the oven.

8. Slice the sweet potatoes lengthwise to open them up.

9. Top with the beans, then the broccoli.

10. Drizzle with the tahini dressing. Season with pepper.

11. Serve the sweet potatoes warm, garnished with the scallions.

SUBSTITUTION TIP: In place of the broccoli, beet greens or Swiss chard work well with the sweet potatoes and black beans. Steam a bunch of either, chopped, in a pot with about ½ inch of water, covered, until tender. Serve alongside the sweet potato and beans.

Per Serving: Calories: 368; Total fat: 15g; Saturated fat: 2g; Sodium: 564mg; Carbohydrates: 52g; Fiber: 14g; Protein: 13g; Calcium: 190mg

Chickpea Veggie Sauté

30 MINUTES OR LESS ∘ ONE POT ∘ VEGAN ∘ VEGETARIAN

Serves 4 / Prep time: 5 minutes / Cook time: 15 minutes

Curry powder is a popular mixture of spices that typically includes turmeric, cumin, coriander, ginger, and pepper and can range from mild to spicy. Use your favorite variety, and adjust the amount as needed depending on the spice level, or add a bit of ground cayenne if you want to heat things up a little more.

- 2 tablespoons extra-virgin olive oil
- 3 garlic cloves, minced
- 1 (15-ounce) can low-sodium chickpeas, drained and rinsed
- 1 (15-ounce) can low-sodium diced tomatoes
- 1 teaspoon curry powder
- ½ teaspoon salt
- ¼ teaspoon freshly ground black pepper
- 4 cups baby spinach

1. In a large skillet, heat the oil over medium heat.

2. Add the garlic, and cook for 30 seconds, or until fragrant.

3. Add the chickpeas, tomatoes with their juices, curry powder, salt, and pepper. Bring to a simmer. Cook, stirring regularly, for about 10 minutes, or until the flavors meld.

4. Add the spinach, and stir for 1 to 2 minutes, or until wilted. Remove from the heat.

FLAVOR BOOST: This is a delicious low-fat curry, but if you want to make a creamy curry, it is really good with ½ cup of coconut milk stirred into the sauce when the spinach is added.

Per Serving: Calories: 168; Total fat: 9g; Saturated fat: 1g; Sodium: 352mg; Carbohydrates: 18g; Fiber: 7g; Protein: 6g; Calcium: 103mg

Chickpea Gyros

30 MINUTES OR LESS ○ ONE POT ○ VEGAN ○ VEGETARIAN

Serves 2 / Prep time: 5 minutes / Cook time: 5 minutes

This vegetarian chickpea gyro has all the flavor of the classic, but instead of beef or lamb, it is stuffed with a simple sautéed chickpea and spice mixture. It is very quick to make on the fly and perfect for a packed lunch. Just be sure to store the tzatziki separately and drizzle it over the pita just before serving.

1 tablespoon extra-virgin olive oil

1 (15-ounce) can low-sodium chickpeas, drained and rinsed

1 teaspoon paprika

½ teaspoon cayenne pepper

2 whole-wheat pita rounds

¼ cup Tzatziki (page 140)

1. In a large skillet, heat the oil over medium heat.

2. Add the chickpeas, and sauté for 2 to 3 minutes, or until heated through.

3. Sprinkle with the paprika and cayenne. Mix well. Cook for 30 seconds, or until fragrant. Remove from the heat.

4. Divide the chickpeas between the pitas.

5. Top with the tzatziki.

FLAVOR BOOST: Add sliced cucumber, lettuce, red onion slices, and tomatoes to the gyros.

Per Serving: Calories: 168; Total fat: 6g; Saturated fat: 1g; Sodium: 262mg; Carbohydrates: 23g; Fiber: 5g; Protein: 6g; Calcium: 68mg

Portabella Mushroom Gyros

30 MINUTES OR LESS ○ ONE POT ○ VEGETARIAN

Serves 4 / Prep time: 5 minutes / Cook time: 10 minutes

Portabella mushrooms soak up any flavor you cook them with, and like all mushrooms, they are a good source of soluble fiber and micronutrients and can help fight cell damage and support bone health. This soy sauce and paprika combination is a savory filling for these umami-packed vegetarian gyros. Look for whole-wheat pita rounds, if available, for the best effects on blood sugar.

2 tablespoons extra-virgin olive oil

4 portabella mushrooms, sliced

1 tablespoon low-sodium soy sauce

½ teaspoon paprika

4 whole-wheat pita rounds

½ cup Tzatziki (page 140)

1. In a skillet, heat the oil over medium-high heat.

2. Add the mushrooms, and sauté for 5 to 7 minutes, or until tender.

3. Turn off the heat. Add the soy sauce and paprika. Stir continuously for about 30 seconds to mix as the soy sauce simmers away in the residual heat of the skillet.

4. Divide the mushrooms among the pitas.

5. Drizzle with the tzatziki.

FLAVOR BOOST: Radishes, cucumber, red onion slices, and lettuce are great additions to these gyros.

Per Serving: Calories: 179; Total fat: 10g; Saturated fat: 1g; Sodium: 350mg; Carbohydrates: 21g; Fiber: 3g; Protein: 6g; Calcium: 72mg

Mujaddara

VEGAN ○ VEGETARIAN

Serves 6 / Prep time: 10 minutes / Cook time: 40 minutes

This simple dish of lentils and rice has been served throughout the Middle East for hundreds of years. It is prepared in various ways depending on where it is served, but typically contains rice and lentils topped with crispy fried onions, which bring loads of flavor.

5 cups water

1 teaspoon salt, divided

1 cup brown basmati rice

1 cup dried brown lentils

¼ cup extra-virgin olive oil

2 large onions, thinly sliced

½ cup chopped fresh parsley

6 scallions, green and white parts, sliced, divided

Freshly ground black pepper

1. In a large saucepan, bring the water and ¾ teaspoon of salt to a boil over high heat.

2. Add the rice, and cook for 10 minutes, lowering the heat to maintain a simmer.

3. Add the lentils, and return to a simmer. Cover the saucepan, and simmer over medium-low heat for 20 to 25 minutes, or until the lentils and rice are tender. Remove from the heat. Drain any remaining liquid. Let rest for 10 minutes.

4. Meanwhile, in a large skillet, heat the oil over medium-high heat. Line a plate with paper towels.

5. Once the oil is hot, add the onions, and cook, stirring regularly, for 20 to 25 minutes, or until well browned. Remove from the heat. Using a slotted spoon, transfer the onions to the prepared plate. Sprinkle with the remaining ¼ teaspoon of salt.

continued

6. Gently mix half of the onions, the parsley, and half of the scallions into the lentils and rice, reserving the remaining onions and scallions for garnish.

7. Serve the lentils and rice topped with the reserved onions and scallions. Season with pepper.

FLAVOR BOOST: Serve the mujaddara with a couple tablespoons of plain yogurt, or to keep it vegan, serve with a side of Garlic Hummus (page 141) or Baba Ghanoush (page 142).

Per Serving: Calories: 333; Total fat: 10g; Saturated fat: 7g; Sodium: 399mg; Carbohydrates: 50g; Fiber: 6g; Protein: 11g; Calcium: 48mg

Eggplant and Chickpea Stew

VEGAN ∘ VEGETARIAN

Serves 6 / Prep time: 15 minutes / Cook time: 50 minutes

Eggplant has a meaty texture and picks up the flavors of whatever it is cooked with, making it the perfect addition to vegan soups and stews. Be sure not to skip the first salting step, which draws the water out of the eggplant and prevents the cooked eggplant in the finished stew from being soggy. Serve the stew with crusty bread and a salad for a more balanced meal!

1½ pounds eggplant, diced

½ teaspoon salt, divided

2 tablespoons extra-virgin olive oil

1 onion, chopped

2 (15-ounce) cans low-sodium chickpeas, drained and rinsed

1 (28-ounce) can low-sodium diced tomatoes

2 cups water, plus more as needed

2 teaspoons paprika

½ teaspoon freshly ground black pepper

Crusty bread, for serving

1. Put the eggplant in a colander, and sprinkle with ¼ teaspoon of salt. Let rest for 10 minutes, then press to extract as much water as possible.

2. In a large pot, heat the oil over medium-high heat.

3. Add the onion, and sauté for 3 to 5 minutes, or until browned.

4. Add the eggplant, chickpeas, tomatoes with their juices, water, paprika, pepper, and remaining ¼ teaspoon of salt.

5. Reduce the heat to medium-low. Cover the pot, and simmer for 30 to 45 minutes, or until the eggplant is tender. Open the lid and stir the mixture a couple times as it cooks, adding more water, ½ cup at a time, to form a sauce. Remove from the heat.

Per Serving: Calories: 206; Total fat: 7g; Saturated fat: 1g; Sodium: 365mg; Carbohydrates: 31g; Fiber: 10g; Protein: 8g; Calcium: 62mg

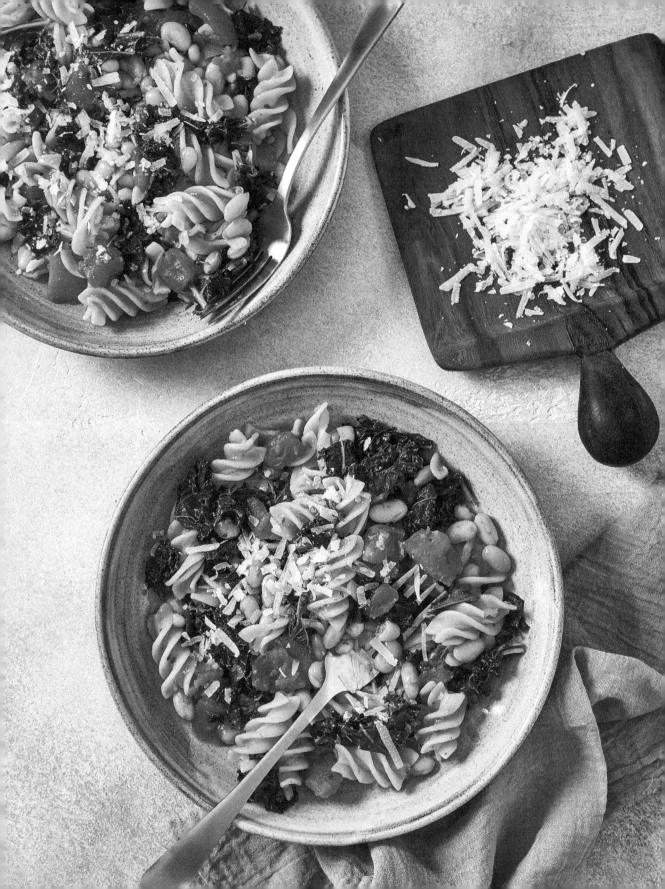

Pasta e Fagioli

30 MINUTES OR LESS ◦ VEGAN ◦ VEGETARIAN

Serves 4 / Prep time: 10 minutes / Cook time: 15 minutes

This pasta and bean dish is teeming with flavor and is done in less than 30 minutes, making it a good weeknight dish. When using canned items like beans and tomatoes, always buy the more heart-healthy low-sodium varieties when available, then adjust the seasoning to your taste.

8 ounces rotini pasta

2 tablespoons extra-virgin olive oil

1 bunch kale, stemmed and chopped

1 (15-ounce) can low-sodium diced tomatoes, drained

1 (15-ounce) can low-sodium white beans, drained and rinsed

1 teaspoon dried oregano

Salt

Freshly ground black pepper

1. Fill a large saucepan with water. Bring to a boil.

2. Cook the pasta according to the package directions, until al dente. Remove from the heat. Reserve about $\frac{1}{2}$ cup of the cooking water, then drain.

3. In a large skillet, heat the oil over medium-high heat.

4. Add the kale, and sauté for 4 to 6 minutes, or until wilted.

5. Add the tomatoes and beans. Cook for 3 to 5 minutes, or until heated through and the tomatoes release some of their water.

6. Season with the oregano, salt, and pepper.

continued

7. Stir the pasta into the skillet along with ¼ cup of the cooking water. Continue cooking, stirring continuously, for 1 more minute, or until heated through. If desired, add the remaining ¼ cup of the cooking water to create a thinner sauce. Remove from the heat.

FLAVOR BOOST: Add 2 tablespoons of shredded Parmesan cheese or vegan shredded "Parmesan" cheese to each serving.

Per Serving: Calories: 435; Total fat: 9g; Saturated fat: 1g; Sodium: 208mg; Carbohydrates: 73g; Fiber: 10g; Protein: 18g; Calcium: 179mg

Cauliflower Shawarma with Tahini

VEGAN ○ VEGETARIAN

Serves 4 / Prep time: 5 minutes / Cook time: 30 minutes

Shawarma is typically made with meats like lamb, beef, or veal and loads of spices, but this stripped-down version uses a mix of paprika, cumin, and coriander to create shawarma cauliflower. Serve this vegan shawarma over Lemon Rice (page 49) or brown rice, or stuff it in a pita.

1 head cauliflower, cut into florets

2 tablespoons extra-virgin olive oil

½ teaspoon ground coriander

1 teaspoon ground cumin

2 teaspoons paprika

Salt

Freshly ground black pepper

½ cup Tahini Dressing (page 145)

1. Preheat the oven to 400°F. Line a baking sheet with parchment paper.

2. In a large bowl, toss together the cauliflower, oil, coriander, cumin, and paprika. Season lightly with salt and pepper.

3. Spread the cauliflower out in a single layer on the prepared baking sheet.

4. Transfer the baking sheet to the oven, and bake for 25 to 30 minutes, or until the cauliflower is tender. Remove from the oven.

5. Drizzle with the dressing.

FLAVOR BOOST: Serve the shawarma topped with finely chopped tomatoes and cucumbers.

Per Serving: Calories: 229; Total fat: 18g; Saturated fat: 2g; Sodium: 314mg; Carbohydrates: 54g; Fiber: 5g; Protein: 7g; Calcium: 170mg

Spaghetti Squash Stuffed with Kale, Artichokes, and Chickpeas

VEGAN ○ VEGETARIAN

Serves 4 / Prep time: 10 minutes / Cook time: 50 minutes

Spaghetti squash has a mild flavor and a texture similar to thin glass noodles when cooked, making it a nice alternative to traditional wheat noodles. Featuring kale, artichoke hearts, and chickpeas, this is a filling dish. Artichoke hearts are loaded with glutathione, a powerful antioxidant, and are one of the most antioxidant-rich vegetables.

2 small spaghetti squash

1 cup water

2 tablespoons extra-virgin olive oil

2 cups chopped kale

1 cup chopped artichoke hearts

1 cup canned chickpeas, drained and rinsed

¼ teaspoon salt

¼ teaspoon freshly ground black pepper

1 cup Marinara Sauce (page 143)

1. Preheat the oven to 400°F.

2. Cut the squash in half lengthwise, and using a spoon, remove the seeds.

3. Place the squash pieces, cut-side down, in a large baking dish.

4. Add the water to the dish, and cover with aluminum foil.

5. Transfer the baking dish to the oven, and bake for 35 to 40 minutes, or until the squash is easily pierced with a fork. Remove from the oven, leaving the oven on.

6. Meanwhile, in a skillet, heat the oil over medium heat.

7. Add the kale, and sauté for 2 to 3 minutes, or until wilted.

8. Add the artichoke hearts and chickpeas. Cook for 2 minutes, or until heated through. Remove from the heat.

9. Using a fork, scrape the flesh from the squash to remove it in strands. Save the squash shells.

10. Mix the strands of spaghetti squash with the vegetable and bean mixture. Season with the salt and pepper. Spoon the mixture back into the squash shell.

11. Drizzle each squash piece with ¼ cup of marinara sauce.

12. Return the baking dish to the oven, and bake for 10 minutes, or until everything is heated through. Remove from the oven.

MAKE IT EASIER: Cook the spaghetti squash on a steam rack in an electric pressure cooker with 1 cup of water on high pressure for 7 minutes. Allow the pressure to release naturally for 10 minutes, then quick-release the remaining pressure.

Per Serving: Calories: 252; Total fat: 13g; Saturated fat: 2g; Sodium: 330mg; Carbohydrates: 32g; Fiber: 10g; Protein: 7g; Calcium: 110mg

Feta and Black Bean–Stuffed Zucchini

VEGETARIAN

Serves 4 / Prep time: 10 minutes / Cook time: 25 minutes

Zucchini is a prolific summer squash that is highly versatile as a low-carb pasta alternative, and in this case, it is stuffed with a delicious black bean, tomato, feta, and mint filling. Because zucchini is not super flavorful on its own, this simple protein-dense filling pairs well with the mild flavor of the squash.

4 medium zucchini, halved lengthwise

2 tablespoons extra-virgin olive oil, divided

1 (15-ounce) can black beans, drained and rinsed

1 large tomato, chopped

½ cup crumbled feta cheese

¼ cup chopped fresh mint leaves

Salt

Freshly ground black pepper

1. Preheat the oven to 400°F.

2. Using a spoon, remove the center of each zucchini, leaving about ½ inch of zucchini skin and flesh. Reserve the flesh.

3. Rub the halved zucchini all over with 1 tablespoon of oil.

4. Place the zucchini, cut-side down, on a baking sheet.

5. Transfer the baking sheet to the oven, and bake for 15 minutes, or until the zucchini is just tender. Remove from the oven, leaving the oven on. Flip the zucchini over so the cut side is up.

6. Meanwhile, chop the reserved zucchini flesh.

7. In a skillet, heat the remaining 1 tablespoon of oil over medium heat.

8. Add the chopped zucchini, and cook for 1 to 2 minutes, or until tender.

9. Add the beans and tomato, and cook for 3 to 5 minutes, or until heated through and the tomato has released its juices.

10. Stir in the cheese and mint. Remove from the heat. Season with salt and pepper.

11. Divide the filling among the zucchini.

12. Return the baking sheet to the oven, and bake for 10 minutes, or until the filling has lightly browned. Remove from the oven.

FLAVOR BOOST: Add 1 chopped chipotle pepper in adobo sauce to the mixture in step 9 for a little added smoky heat.

Per Serving: Calories: 236; Total fat: 12g; Saturated fat: 4g; Sodium: 229mg; Carbohydrates: 24g; Fiber: 8g; Protein: 11g; Calcium: 146mg

Spiced Lentils

30 MINUTES OR LESS ∘ VEGAN ∘ VEGETARIAN

Serves 4 / Prep time: 10 minutes / Cook time: 20 minutes

Lentils are so versatile—they can be used in soups, stews, sautés, and snacks. Here they are pan-fried with pureed onion and bell pepper for a flavorful main course dish. Serve them over rice, or scoop them up with pieces of naan, flatbread, or pita.

2 cups water

1 cup dried green or brown lentils

1 large onion, coarsely chopped

1 large red bell pepper, chopped

1 tablespoon paprika

½ teaspoon cayenne pepper

½ teaspoon salt, plus more as needed

¼ teaspoon freshly ground black pepper, plus more as needed

2 tablespoons extra-virgin olive oil

1. In a large saucepan, combine the water and lentils. Bring to a boil.

2. Reduce the heat to a simmer. Cook for 20 minutes, or until the lentils are tender but still holding their shape. Remove from the heat. Drain any remaining liquid.

3. Meanwhile, in a food processor or blender, combine the onion, bell pepper, paprika, cayenne, ½ teaspoon of salt, and ¼ teaspoon black pepper. Process into a puree.

4. In a large skillet, heat the oil over medium-high heat.

5. Add the onion–bell pepper mixture, and cook for 2 to 3 minutes, or until lightly browned and fragrant.

6. Add the lentils, and toss well. Remove from the heat. Season with additional salt and pepper.

Per Serving: Calories: 262; Total fat: 8g; Saturated fat: 1g; Sodium: 298mg; Carbohydrates: 37g; Fiber: 7g; Protein: 13g; Calcium: 33mg

Basil-Bean Salad

ONE POT ○ VEGAN ○ VEGETARIAN

Serves 4 / Prep time: 10 minutes + 1 hour to chill

This salad comes together in minutes and is incredibly versatile, so feel free to get creative with additional vegetables. Cucumber brings a little crunch, and basil and lemon vinaigrette tie it all together. Because the cornerstone of the salad is beans, this is a good main course meal, especially when paired with a Simple Green Salad (page 37).

1 (15-ounce) can low-sodium kidney beans, drained and rinsed

1 (15-ounce) can low-sodium chickpeas, drained and rinsed

1 English cucumber, finely diced

½ cup Lemon Vinaigrette (page 148)

¼ cup thinly sliced fresh basil leaves

In a large bowl, toss together the kidney beans, chickpeas, cucumber, vinaigrette, and basil. Refrigerate for 1 hour before serving to allow the flavors to meld.

SUBSTITUTION TIP: Balsamic Vinaigrette (page 147) or Tahini Dressing (page 145) can both be used in place of Lemon Vinaigrette in this recipe.

Per Serving: Calories: 357; Total fat: 20g; Saturated fat: 2g; Sodium: 348mg; Carbohydrates: 34g; Fiber: 8g; Protein: 10g; Calcium: 68mg

Fried Eggplant, Zucchini, and Tomatoes

30 MINUTES OR LESS ○ VEGAN ○ VEGETARIAN

Serves 4 / Prep time: 10 minutes / Cook time: 20 minutes

Za'atar, a Mediterranean and Middle Eastern spice blend consisting of sesame seeds, sumac, and a blend of thyme, oregano, and marjoram, flavors this trio of vegetables for a simple and quick meal. This vegetable dish is great over brown rice or stuffed into a pita.

3 tablespoons extra-virgin olive oil

1 teaspoon za'atar

1 large eggplant, sliced lengthwise

2 medium zucchini, sliced lengthwise

2 large tomatoes, sliced

Salt

Freshly ground black pepper

½ cup Garlic Hummus (page 141)

1. In a small bowl, mix together the oil and za'atar.

2. Heat a large skillet or grill pan over medium heat. Line a large plate with paper towels.

3. Season the eggplant, zucchini, and tomatoes with salt and pepper.

4. Brush the eggplant slices on both sides with about 1 tablespoon of the za'atar oil. Put them in the skillet, and cook, flipping once, for 4 to 5 minutes per side, or until browned and tender. Remove from the skillet. Transfer to the prepared plate.

5. Brush the zucchini with about 1 tablespoon of the za'atar oil. Put them in the skillet, and cook, flipping once, for 2 to 3 minutes per side, or until browned and tender. Transfer to the prepared plate.

6. Brush the tomatoes with the remaining za'atar oil. Put them in the skillet, and cook for 2 to 3 minutes per side, or until lightly browned and heated through. Remove from the heat.

7. Serve the vegetables topped with the hummus.

FLAVOR BOOST: Serve topped with 2 tablespoons of chopped parsley or cilantro.

Per Serving: Calories: 211; Total fat: 14g; Saturated fat: 2g; Sodium: 129mg; Carbohydrates: 21g; Fiber: 7g; Protein: 5g; Calcium: 52mg

Eggplant Caponata

VEGAN ○ VEGETARIAN

Serves 4 / Prep time: 10 minutes / Cook time: 30 minutes

This tomato-eggplant sauce can replace your meaty spaghetti sauce for a lightened-up vegan alternative. The purple-black skin of the eggplant contains anthocyanin, which has been shown to lower blood pressure. Serve the finished sauce over whole-wheat pasta or zucchini noodles, or sop it up with crusty bread.

1 large eggplant, cut into ½-inch dice

Salt

3 tablespoons extra-virgin olive oil

1 onion, chopped

1 (15-ounce) can diced tomatoes with Italian seasonings

¼ cup chopped pitted green olives

2 tablespoons red-wine vinegar

Freshly ground black pepper

1. In a colander, toss the eggplant with a couple pinches of salt. Let rest for 10 minutes.

2. In a skillet, heat the oil over medium-high heat.

3. Add the onion, and cook for 3 to 5 minutes, or until softened.

4. Squeeze out any water accumulated on the eggplant. Add the eggplant to the skillet. Cook for 10 to 15 minutes, or until browned and tender.

5. Add the tomatoes with their juices, olives, and vinegar. Simmer for about 10 minutes, or until the flavors meld and the sauce thickens. Remove from the heat. Season with salt and pepper.

FLAVOR BOOST: Top with 2 tablespoons of shredded Parmesan cheese and 2 tablespoons of chopped fresh parsley and mint per serving.

Per Serving: Calories: 165; Total fat: 12g; Saturated fat: 2g; Sodium: 110mg; Carbohydrates: 15g; Fiber: 6g; Protein: 3g; Calcium: 37mg

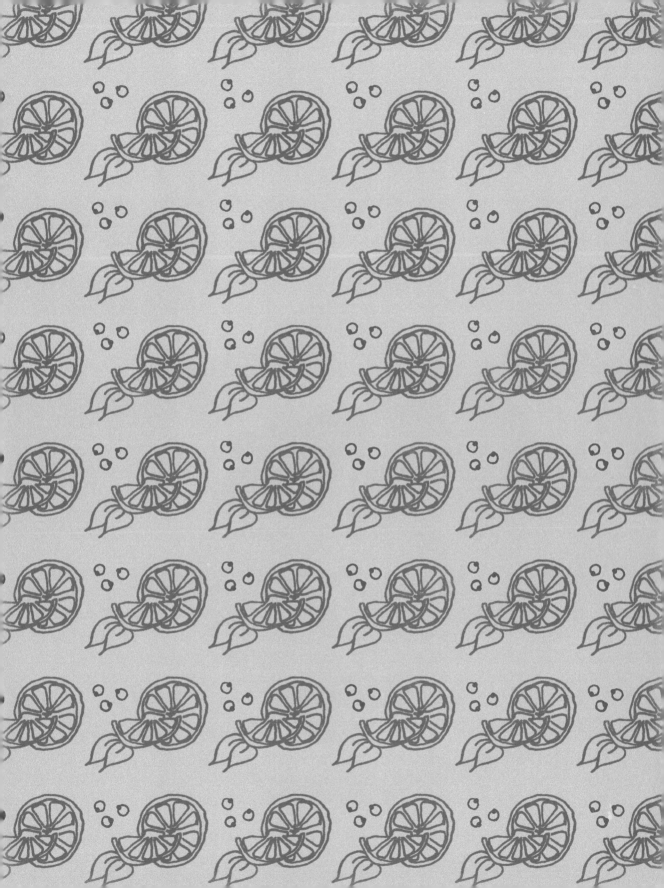

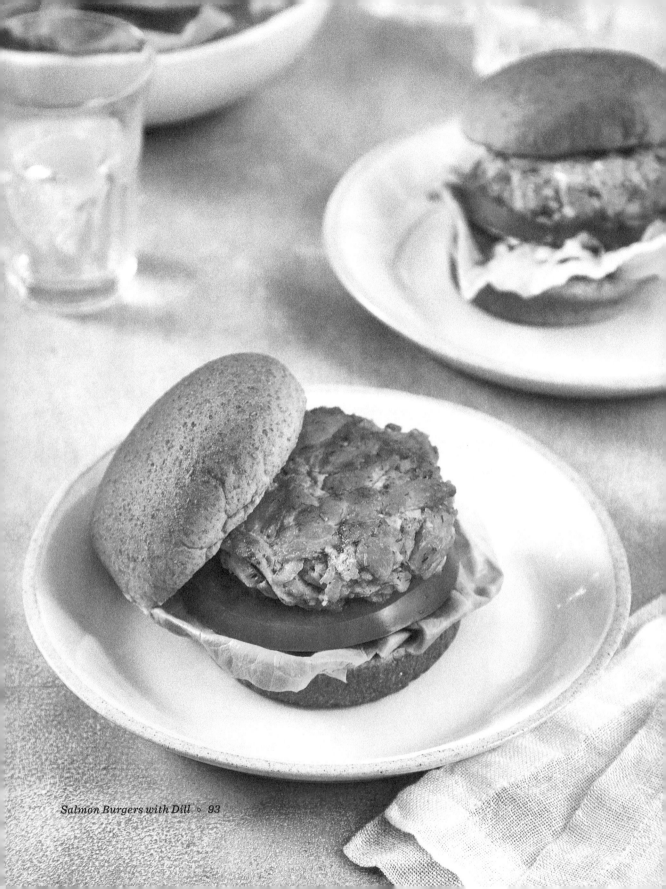

Salmon Burgers with Dill ○ 93

CHAPTER FIVE

Fish and Seafood Mains

Chickpea Salad with Tuna

30 MINUTES OR LESS ∘ ONE POT

Serves 4 / Prep time: 10 minutes

Chickpeas and tuna combine in this quick salad perfect for a workday lunch or easy dinner. Requiring no cooking, this salad is fresh and loaded with omega-3s from the tuna, and fiber, iron, magnesium, and B vitamins from the chickpeas, all of which support heart health. The salad is hearty on its own but can be served over a bed of salad greens if desired.

1 English cucumber, chopped

1 (15-ounce) can chickpeas, drained and rinsed

2 (5-ounce) cans water-packed tuna, drained

½ red onion, sliced

¼ cup Lemon Vinaigrette (page 148)

1. In a large bowl, toss together the cucumber, chickpeas, tuna, and onion.

2. Drizzle with the vinaigrette, and toss to combine. Serve at room temperature or cold.

FLAVOR BOOST: Add 2 tablespoons of chopped fresh dill to the salad.

Per Serving: Calories: 234; Total fat: 11g; Saturated fat: 1g; Sodium: 375mg; Carbohydrates: 18g; Fiber: 4g; Protein: 16g; Calcium: 52mg

Avocado and Tuna Salad Sandwich

30 MINUTES OR LESS ○ ONE POT

Serves 2 / Prep time: 10 minutes

Avocado is a creamy alternative to mayonnaise in this tuna salad sandwich. Avocado is rich in monounsaturated fats, as well as B vitamins, fiber, and vitamin E, making it a heart-healthy substitute for mayonnaise. Here the avocado is cut into pieces and mixed, but if you prefer a creamier salad, you can mash the avocado to create a texture similar to a traditional tuna salad.

1 (5-ounce) can water-packed tuna, drained

1 ripe avocado, pitted, peeled, and chopped

2 scallions, green and white parts, minced

Juice of ½ lemon

2 tablespoons extra-virgin olive oil

¼ teaspoon salt

¼ teaspoon freshly ground black pepper

4 whole-wheat bread slices

1. In a small bowl, combine the tuna, avocado, scallions, lemon juice, oil, salt, and pepper.

2. Divide the tuna mixture onto 2 bread slices. Top with the remaining 2 bread slices.

FLAVOR BOOST: Add a couple teaspoons of chopped fresh cilantro or parsley to the tuna salad if desired, or for a little more texture, add ¼ cup of finely chopped celery.

Per Serving: Calories: 518; Total fat: 32g; Saturated fat: 5g; Sodium: 567mg; Carbohydrates: 41g; Fiber: 13g; Protein: 23g; Calcium: 140mg

Salmon over Lentils

30 MINUTES OR LESS

Serves 4 / Prep time: 5 minutes / Cook time: 25 minutes

Salmon and lentils are a wonderful heart-healthy pair. Salmon is rich in omega-3 fatty acids, and lentils contain a mix of magnesium, calcium, and potassium, all of which combine to help reduce the risk of heart disease. This is a filling meal on its own, but it also pairs nicely with any leafy green salad.

1 cup dried brown lentils

4 (4-ounce) salmon fillets

½ teaspoon salt, divided

¼ teaspoon freshly ground black pepper

2 tablespoons extra-virgin olive oil

1 onion, chopped

1 carrot, finely chopped

1 teaspoon dried thyme

1. Preheat the oven to 400°F. Line a baking sheet with parchment paper.

2. In a large saucepan, cover the lentils with water by about 2 inches. Bring to a boil.

3. Reduce the heat to low. Simmer for 20 minutes, or until the lentils are just tender but not mushy. Remove from the heat. Drain.

4. While the lentils are cooking, put the salmon on the prepared baking sheet. Season with ¼ teaspoon of salt and the pepper.

5. Transfer the baking sheet to the oven, and bake for 15 to 20 minutes, or until the salmon flakes easily with a fork. Remove from the oven.

6. In a skillet, heat the oil over medium-high heat.

7. Add the onion and carrot. Sauté for 3 to 5 minutes, or until just softened.

8. Add the thyme and remaining $\frac{1}{4}$ teaspoon of salt.

9. Stir in the lentils, and mix well. Remove from the heat.

10. Serve the salmon fillets on a bed of lentils.

SUBSTITUTION TIP: One tablespoon of chopped fresh dill works well in this recipe in place of the thyme.

Per Serving: Calories: 407; Total fat: 15g; Saturated fat: 2g; Sodium: 355mg; Carbohydrates: 34g; Fiber: 6g; Protein: 35g; Calcium: 43mg

Salmon and Chickpeas with Arugula

Serves 4 / Prep time: 5 minutes / Cook time: 25 minutes

Canned chickpeas are convenient for adding fiber to your diet without the work of soaking and cooking them. In this quick recipe, the fiber-rich chickpeas are mixed with arugula and cumin and topped with salmon. The lemon vinaigrette ties everything together and brings a burst of vitamin C to finish the dish.

4 (4-ounce) salmon fillets

2 tablespoons extra-virgin olive oil, divided

¼ teaspoon salt

¼ teaspoon freshly ground black pepper

1 (15-ounce) can chickpeas, drained and rinsed

½ teaspoon ground cumin

4 cups arugula

¼ cup Lemon Vinaigrette (page 148)

1. Preheat the oven to 400°F. Line a baking sheet with parchment paper.

2. Put the salmon fillets on the prepared baking sheet.

3. Drizzle the salmon with 1 tablespoon of oil. Season with the salt and pepper.

4. Transfer the baking sheet to the oven, and bake for 16 to 20 minutes, or until the salmon has cooked through and flakes easily with a fork. Remove from the oven.

5. In a large skillet, heat the remaining 1 tablespoon of oil over medium-high heat.

6. Add the chickpeas and cumin. Cook for 2 to 3 minutes, or until heated through. Remove from the heat.

7. Mix in the arugula until wilted.

8. Serve the salmon atop the chickpeas and arugula, drizzled with the vinaigrette.

Per Serving: Calories: 395; Total fat: 25g; Saturated fat: 3g; Sodium: 442mg; Carbohydrates: 15g; Fiber: 4g; Protein: 27g; Calcium: 76mg

Salmon Burgers with Dill

Serves 4 / Prep time: 5 minutes / Cook time: 35 minutes

Salmon burgers are a great way to get your omega-3s, and these easy-to-make burgers are just the thing for a weeknight meal. Seasoned with dill, which is rich in heart-healthy flavonoids, these simple burgers will liven up your meal routine. Serve the burgers on whole-wheat buns or over a salad for a light meal.

1 pound salmon fillets

½ teaspoon salt, divided

¼ teaspoon freshly ground black pepper

½ cup bread crumbs

1 large egg

2 garlic cloves, minced

½ teaspoon dried dill

2 tablespoons extra-virgin olive oil

1. Preheat the oven to 400°F. Line a baking sheet with parchment paper.

2. Put the salmon on the prepared baking sheet. Season with ¼ teaspoon of salt and the pepper.

3. Transfer the baking sheet to the oven, and bake for 15 to 20 minutes, or until the salmon flakes with a fork. Remove from the oven.

4. Remove the salmon flesh from the skin. Transfer the flesh to a bowl, removing any bones.

5. Mix in the bread crumbs, egg, garlic, dill, and remaining ¼ teaspoon of salt.

6. Form the mixture into 4 patties.

7. In a large skillet, heat the oil over medium heat.

8. Add the patties, and cook for 5 to 6 minutes, or until browned. Flip, and cook on the other side for 3 to 5 minutes. Remove from the heat.

Per Serving: Calories: 294; Total fat: 16g; Saturated fat: 3g; Sodium: 458mg; Carbohydrates: 10g; Fiber: 1g; Protein: 26g; Calcium: 51mg

Whole Branzino

Serves 2 / Prep time: 5 minutes / Cook time: 25 minutes

Branzino is a light and flaky fish with a mild, sweet flavor and is popular through-out the Mediterranean. It is perfect for serving two people, because its large meaty fillets can be removed easily. Rich in protein and the antioxidant selenium, branzino is a heart-healthy choice.

4 garlic cloves, peeled

2 thyme sprigs

1 oregano sprig

1 whole branzino, dressed and rinsed

2 lemons, sliced, divided

¼ teaspoon salt

¼ teaspoon freshly ground black pepper

1. Preheat the oven to 450°F.

2. Place the garlic, thyme, and oregano inside the branzino.

3. Place half of the lemon slices inside the branzino. Season the outside with the salt and pepper.

4. Put the branzino on a baking sheet.

5. Transfer the baking sheet to the oven, and roast for 18 to 22 minutes, or until the branzino has cooked through. Remove from the oven.

6. Fillet the branzino, and serve with the remaining lemon slices.

FLAVOR BOOST: Serve the branzino topped with ¼ cup of chopped fresh parsley.

Per Serving: Calories: 218; Total fat: 3g; Saturated fat: 1g; Sodium: 430mg; Carbohydrates: 0g; Fiber: 0g; Protein: 45g; Calcium: 70mg

Baked Halibut Steaks

30 MINUTES OR LESS ◦ ONE POT

Serves 4 / Prep time: 5 minutes / Cook time: 15 minutes

Halibut is a light, clean-tasting fish. Za'atar and lemon provide the dominant flavor here, and these steaks are baked in the oven to make prep simple. If you have a little extra time to get the grill heated, halibut steaks are also great when cooked over a medium-high grill for the same amount of time.

4 (4-ounce) halibut steaks

2 tablespoons extra-virgin olive oil

1 teaspoon za'atar

½ teaspoon salt

¼ teaspoon freshly ground black pepper

1 lemon, cut into wedges

2 tablespoons chopped fresh parsley

1. Preheat the oven to 400°F. Line a baking sheet with parchment paper.

2. Put the halibut on the prepared baking sheet.

3. Drizzle with the oil.

4. Season both sides with the za'atar, salt, and pepper.

5. Transfer the baking sheet to the oven, and bake for 6 to 8 minutes. Flip, then cook for 5 minutes, or until the halibut has cooked through and flakes easily with a fork. Remove from the oven.

6. Serve the halibut topped with the lemon wedges and parsley.

SUBSTITUTION TIP: Any number of spices make a good substitute for the za'atar. Try this sprinkled with ground cumin or paprika instead.

Per Serving: Calories: 164; Total fat: 8g; Saturated fat: 1g; Sodium: 369mg; Carbohydrates: 0g; Fiber: 0g; Protein: 21g; Calcium: 11mg

Walnut-and-Herb–Crusted Fish

Serves 4 / Prep time: 5 minutes / Cook time: 20 minutes

Walnuts, herbs, and Parmesan cheese form a great breading on fish when ground finely in a food processor to resemble bread crumbs. This technique works great on mild white fish but can also be used on fatty fish like salmon and trout. Breading and baking fish is a great way to replace fried fish in your diet.

¼ cup chopped walnuts

¼ cup shredded
  Parmesan cheese

2 tablespoons chopped
  fresh parsley

1 tablespoon chopped fresh
  basil leaves

1 pound sole or tilapia fillets

2 tablespoons extra-virgin
  olive oil

¼ teaspoon salt

¼ teaspoon freshly ground
  black pepper

1. Preheat the oven to 400°F.

2. In a food processor, combine the walnuts and cheese. Process until it forms crumbs.

3. Add the parsley and basil. Pulse until the mixture is combined.

4. Put the fillets on a baking sheet.

5. Brush the fillets with the oil. Season with the salt and pepper.

6. Press the walnut and cheese mixture into the fillets.

7. Transfer the baking sheet to the oven, and bake for 15 to 20 minutes, or until the fillets have cooked through and flake easily with a fork and the breading has browned. Remove from the oven.

Per Serving: Calories: 244; Total fat: 15g; Saturated fat: 3g; Sodium: 338mg; Carbohydrates: 2g; Fiber: 1g; Protein: 21g; Calcium: 76mg

Cod Parcels with Mushrooms and Spinach

Cooking fish enclosed in a packet locks in the juices, making it moist and tender. Mushrooms are rich in vitamin D and can help lower cholesterol, making them a good option for heart health. This low-fat fish dish is a light meal on its own or can be combined with Lemon Rice (page 49) or Quinoa Tabbouleh (page 50) for a heartier meal.

4 cups baby spinach

2 cups sliced shiitake mushrooms

4 (4-ounce) cod fillets

½ teaspoon Old Bay seasoning

½ teaspoon salt

¼ teaspoon freshly ground black pepper

¼ cup chopped scallions, green and white parts

2 tablespoons extra-virgin olive oil

1. Preheat the oven to 425°F.

2. Tear 4 (12-inch) square pieces of aluminum foil. Into each piece of foil, place 1 cup of spinach and ½ cup of mushrooms.

3. Place 1 piece of cod on top.

4. Season with the Old Bay, salt, and pepper.

5. Sprinkle with the scallions, and drizzle with the oil.

6. Fold up the packets to seal and enclose the cod.

7. Place the packets on a baking sheet.

8. Transfer the baking sheet to the oven, and bake for 15 minutes. Remove from the oven. Carefully unfold the packets.

Per Serving: Calories: 155; Total fat: 7g; Saturated fat: 1g; Sodium: 435mg; Carbohydrates: 3g; Fiber: 1g; Protein: 19g; Calcium: 45mg

Weeknight Fish Skillet

30 MINUTES OR LESS ○ ONE POT

Serves 4 / Prep time: 5 minutes / Cook time: 20 minutes

A simple fish skillet is quick and easy to throw together, making it a great choice after a long day. Serve it with cauliflower rice or Zucchini Noodles (page 48) for a light and flavorful meal. This skillet will work with any white fish, but you will need to adjust the cooking time as needed to account for the thickness of the fish.

1 pound cod, halibut, or mahi mahi fillets

½ teaspoon salt

¼ teaspoon freshly ground black pepper

1 tablespoon extra-virgin olive oil

1 red bell pepper, cored and chopped

1 red onion, chopped

2 cups cherry tomatoes

¼ cup chopped pitted green olives

1. Season the fillets with the salt and pepper.

2. In a large skillet, heat the oil over medium-high heat.

3. Add the bell pepper and onion. Cook for 3 to 5 minutes, or until softened.

4. Add the tomatoes and olives. Stir for 1 to 2 minutes, or until the tomatoes begin to soften.

5. Nestle the fillets on top of the vegetables, cover the skillet, and cook for 5 to 10 minutes, or until the fillets flake easily with a fork. Remove from the heat.

FLAVOR BOOST: Squeeze the juice from a lemon on top of the fish and vegetables after cooking.

Per Serving: Calories: 151; Total fat: 5g; Saturated fat: 1g; Sodium: 603mg; Carbohydrates: 8g; Fiber: 2g; Protein: 19g; Calcium: 33mg

Broiled Pesto Cod

Serves 4 / Prep time: 5 minutes / Cook time: 25 minutes

Pesto's nutty and rich flavor is great when paired with a mild fish like cod. Cod fillets are typically thin, so this dish is easily ready in 30 minutes. Choose wild-caught cod for the best nutrient profile and sustainability. Although cod contains lower levels of omega-3s than other fattier fishes, it is an excellent lean protein choice that is a great addition to your diet.

1 pound cod fillets	¼ cup Basil-Walnut Pesto (page 144)	1 large tomato, chopped
Salt		
Freshly ground black pepper	2 tablespoons whole-wheat panko bread crumbs	

1. Preheat the oven to 400°F. Line a baking sheet with parchment paper.

2. Put the cod on the prepared baking sheet. Season lightly with salt and pepper.

3. Spread the pesto over the cod in an even layer.

4. Sprinkle the bread crumbs on top.

5. Transfer the baking sheet to the oven, and bake for 16 to 20 minutes, or until the bread crumbs have browned and the cod flakes easily with a fork. Remove from the oven, leaving the oven on.

6. Top the cod with the tomato.

7. Return the baking sheet to the oven, and bake for 2 minutes, or until the tomato is heated through. Remove from the oven.

Per Serving: Calories: 183; Total fat: 9g; Saturated fat: 2g; Sodium: 549mg; Carbohydrates: 5g; Fiber: 1g; Protein: 20g; Calcium: 56mg

Shrimp Paella

Serves 4 / Prep time: 5 minutes / Cook time: 40 minutes

Paella is a one-dish meal that is traditionally cooked in a special paella pan but is easily re-created in a large skillet on the stovetop. Look for any medium-grain rice to best replicate the texture of the traditional dish but with the convenience of this streamlined version.

2 tablespoons extra-virgin olive oil, divided

1 pound large shrimp, peeled and deveined

1 onion, chopped

2 cups medium-grain white rice

3½ cups water

1 (14½-ounce) can low-sodium diced tomatoes, drained

½ teaspoon paprika

¼ teaspoon salt

¼ teaspoon freshly ground black pepper

1. In a large skillet, heat 1 tablespoon of oil over medium-high heat.

2. Add the shrimp, and cook for 2 to 3 minutes per side, or until just cooked through, being careful not to overcook. Transfer to a plate.

3. In the same skillet, heat the remaining 1 tablespoon of oil over medium heat.

4. Add the onion, and cook for 3 to 5 minutes, or until softened.

5. Add the rice, and stir to coat with the oil.

6. Add the water, tomatoes, paprika, salt, and pepper. Bring to a boil.

7. Reduce the heat to a simmer. Cover the skillet, and cook for 20 to 25 minutes, or until the water has been absorbed. Remove from the heat.

8. Stir in the shrimp.

Per Serving: Calories: 519; Total fat: 9g; Saturated fat: 1g; Sodium: 334mg; Carbohydrates: 85g; Fiber: 4g; Protein: 23g; Calcium: 111mg

Shrimp Scampi

30 MINUTES OR LESS ∘ ONE POT
Serves 4 / Prep time: 5 minutes / Cook time: 10 minutes

Shrimp scampi is a classic dish that is a lot easier to make than you may think. Shrimp is a low-calorie, high-protein food source that is rich in omega-3s and low in saturated fat, making it a great addition to your plate. Flavored with lemon juice and garlic, shrimp comes alive in this simple preparation. Serve the scampi with a salad or over a bed of Zucchini Noodles (page 48).

2 tablespoons extra-virgin olive oil

6 garlic cloves, minced

½ cup dry white wine

1 pound shrimp, peeled and deveined

¼ teaspoon salt

Juice of 1 lemon

2 tablespoons chopped fresh parsley

1. In a large skillet, heat the oil over medium-high heat.

2. Add the garlic, and cook for 30 seconds, or until fragrant.

3. Add the wine, and simmer for 2 to 3 minutes, or until reduced by about half.

4. Add the shrimp, and cook for 3 to 5 minutes, or until cooked through and pink. Remove from the heat. Season with the salt.

5. Sprinkle the lemon juice over the shrimp.

6. Garnish with the parsley.

FLAVOR BOOST: Shredded Parmesan cheese is a great addition to scampi. Sprinkle a tablespoon over each serving.

Per Serving: Calories: 190; Total fat: 7g; Saturated fat: 1g; Sodium: 284mg; Carbohydrates: 3g; Fiber: 0g; Protein: 23g; Calcium: 87mg

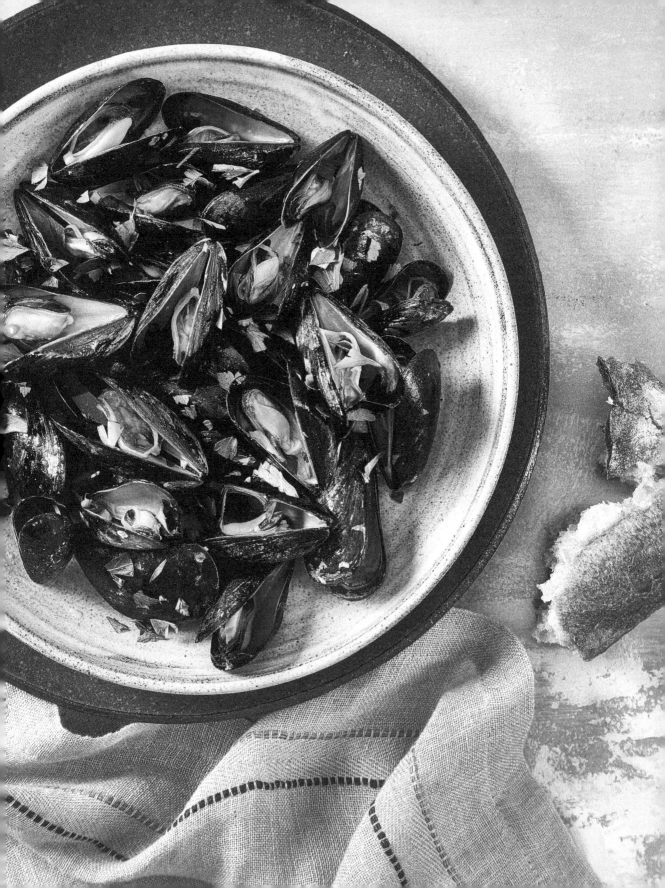

Mussels with White Wine Sauce

30 MINUTES OR LESS

Serves 4 / Prep time: 15 minutes / Cook time: 15 minutes

Mussels are quick cooking and perfect for an easy weeknight meal. They are a great source of vitamins A and B_{12} and are a wonderful source of protein. Serve them with crusty bread to sop up all the delicious juices.

2 pounds mussels

½ cup dry white wine

2 tablespoons extra-virgin olive oil

3 garlic cloves, minced

¼ cup chopped fresh parsley

1. Clean and prep the mussels. Remove any beards.

2. Put the mussels and wine in a large pot. Bring to a boil.

3. Cover the pot, and reduce the heat to low. The mussels will release juices as they cook. Cook for 5 to 7 minutes, or until the mussels have opened. Remove from the heat. Using a slotted spoon, remove the mussels from the pot, leaving the liquid in the pot. Discard any mussels that have not opened.

4. Let the liquid rest for a couple of minutes, then carefully pour the liquid off the top into a small bowl, leaving behind the grit and sediment.

5. In a small saucepan, heat the oil over medium heat.

6. Add the garlic, and sauté for 30 seconds, or until fragrant.

7. Add the cooking liquid, and simmer for 2 to 3 minutes, or until slightly reduced. Remove from the heat.

8. Serve the mussels with the sauce poured over them.

9. Garnish with the parsley.

Per Serving: Calories: 137; Total fat: 8g; Saturated fat: 1g; Sodium: 166mg; Carbohydrates: 4g; Fiber: 0g; Protein: 7g; Calcium: 27mg

Lemon-Rosemary Salmon

Serves 4 / Prep time: 5 minutes / Cook time: 20 minutes

Salmon is a heart-healthy fish that tastes great with so many different flavors, as in this combination of rosemary, lemon, and whole-grain mustard. Choose wild salmon over farm-raised salmon for the most omega-3 fatty acids. Serve on a bed of whole grains, with Israeli Couscous Salad (page 44), or with cauliflower rice.

Zest and juice of ½ lemon

1 tablespoon extra-virgin olive oil

2 teaspoons whole-grain mustard

½ teaspoon dried rosemary

¼ teaspoon salt

¼ teaspoon freshly ground black pepper

1 pound salmon fillets

1. Preheat the oven to 400°F. Line a baking sheet with parchment paper.

2. In a small bowl, combine the lemon zest and juice, oil, mustard, rosemary, salt, and pepper.

3. Put the salmon on the prepared baking sheet.

4. Spread the mixture on the salmon.

5. Transfer the baking sheet to the oven, and bake for 16 to 20 minutes, or until the salmon has cooked through and flakes easily with a fork. Remove from the oven.

SUBSTITUTION TIP: The whole-grain mustard can be substituted with Dijon mustard.

Per Serving: Calories: 194; Total fat: 11g; Saturated fat: 2g; Sodium: 223mg; Carbohydrates: 1g; Fiber: 0g; Protein: 23g; Calcium: 16mg

Pan-Seared Cod with Swiss Chard and Lemon

30 MINUTES OR LESS

Serves 4 / Prep time: 5 minutes / Cook time: 10 minutes

Pan-searing cod creates a nice crust on the fish, and if you pair it with an easy-to-cook green like chard, you can have dinner on the table in minutes. Serve on its own or with Lemon Rice (page 49) or Israeli Couscous Salad (page 44).

3 tablespoons extra-virgin olive oil, divided

2 garlic cloves, minced

1 pound Swiss chard, both leaves and stems, thick stems removed, thinly sliced

4 (4-ounce) cod fillets

¼ teaspoon salt

¼ teaspoon freshly ground black pepper

1 lemon, cut into wedges

1. In a large skillet, heat 1½ tablespoons of oil over medium heat.

2. Add the garlic, and cook for 30 seconds, or until fragrant.

3. Add the chard, and cook, stirring occasionally, for 6 to 8 minutes, or until wilted and tender. Remove from the heat.

4. Meanwhile, in a separate large skillet, heat the remaining 1½ tablespoons of oil over medium-high heat.

5. Season the cod with the salt and pepper. Add the cod to the skillet, and sear for 3 to 5 minutes per side, or until cooked through. Remove from the heat.

6. Serve the cod atop the chard with the lemon wedges on the side.

SUBSTITUTION TIP: Use mustard greens, collard greens, or spinach in place of the chard. Adjust cooking times as needed to cook the greens until tender and wilted.

Per Serving: Calories: 206; Total fat: 11g; Saturated fat: 2g; Sodium: 225mg; Carbohydrates: 5g; Fiber: 2g; Protein: 22g; Calcium: 79mg

Poached Fish in Tomato-Caper Sauce

Serves 4 / Prep time: 5 minutes / Cook time: 30 minutes

Capers bring a flavorful touch to tomato sauce and pair nicely with the mild flavor of cod. Poaching fish in a liquid is a quick way to cook it and keeps it tender and moist. Tomatoes are rich in lycopene, an antioxidant that has been linked to lowering LDL cholesterol and lowering the risk of stroke.

1 (28-ounce) can low-sodium diced tomatoes

¼ cup capers, drained, rinsed, and finely chopped

3 garlic cloves, minced

1 teaspoon paprika

½ teaspoon salt

¼ teaspoon freshly ground black pepper

1 pound cod or halibut fillets

1. In a large saucepan, combine the tomatoes with their juices, capers, garlic, paprika, salt, and pepper. Bring to a simmer over medium heat. Cook, stirring occasionally, for 15 minutes, or until thickened.

2. Using a spatula, slide the fillets into the saucepan, and cook for 10 to 15 minutes, or until they flake easily with a fork. Remove from the heat.

FLAVOR BOOST: Add 1 or 2 tablespoons of chopped thyme or basil to the sauce. If desired, add a pinch of sugar to the sauce to sweeten it.

Per Serving: Calories: 130; Total fat: 1g; Saturated fat: 0g; Sodium: 388mg; Carbohydrates: 8g; Fiber: 4g; Protein: 22g; Calcium: 89mg

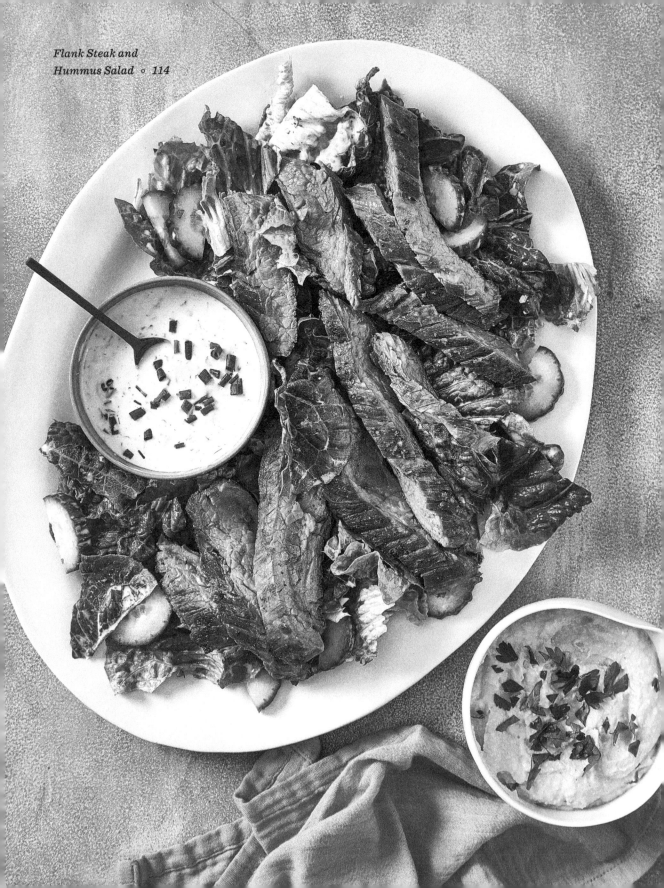

— CHAPTER SIX —

Poultry and Meat Mains

continued

Poultry and Meat Mains

continued

Egg, Lemon, and Chicken Soup

Serves 6 / Prep time: 10 minutes / Cook time: 40 minutes

This hearty soup, also known as avgolemono, is a bright Greek chicken soup. The lemon juice is the standout flavor in this comforting meal. Lemon juice is rich in vitamin C, making this a good immune booster. Here we use homemade vegetable stock, but feel free to substitute store-bought low-sodium chicken or vegetable broth.

8 cups Vegetable Stock (page 150) or store-bought low-sodium broth

8 ounces boneless, skinless chicken breast

1 cup long-grain white rice

2 large eggs

⅓ cup freshly squeezed lemon juice

1 teaspoon grated lemon zest

½ teaspoon salt

¼ teaspoon freshly ground black pepper

1. In a large saucepan, bring the stock to a simmer over medium heat.

2. Add the chicken, and cook for 15 to 20 minutes, or until cooked through. Remove from the heat. Transfer the chicken to a bowl, and set aside to cool. Once cool, using 2 forks, shred.

3. Return the chicken to the stock, and add the rice. Cook over medium heat for 15 minutes, or until tender.

4. Reduce the heat to medium-low.

5. In a small bowl, whisk together the eggs, lemon juice, and lemon zest.

6. While whisking, ladle a cup of the stock into the lemon and egg mixture to temper the sauce.

7. Whisk the egg mixture into the saucepan continuously for about 1 minute, then remove from the heat. Season with the salt and pepper.

Per Serving: Calories: 191; Total fat: 3g; Saturated fat: 1g; Sodium: 235mg; Carbohydrates: 27g; Fiber: 1g; Protein: 13g; Calcium: 13mg

Chicken and Tomato Stew

ONE POT

Serves 4 / Prep time: 5 minutes / Cook time: 30 minutes

This thick and hearty stew is made creamy with the addition of tahini, which is loaded with flavor and health benefits. Tahini, or ground sesame seeds, is rich in lignan, a powerful antioxidant that can help reduce the risk of heart disease and inflammation.

1 tablespoon extra-virgin olive oil

½ onion, finely chopped

8 ounces boneless, skinless chicken breast

2 cups water

1 (15-ounce) can low-sodium diced tomatoes

½ cup quinoa

½ teaspoon salt

¼ teaspoon freshly ground black pepper

½ cup tahini

1. In a large pot, heat the oil over medium heat.

2. Add the onion, and cook for 3 to 5 minutes, or until softened.

3. Add the chicken, and cook, stirring occasionally, for 5 minutes, or until browned.

4. Add the water, tomatoes with their juices, quinoa, salt, and pepper. Simmer for 20 minutes, or until the quinoa is tender.

5. Stir in the tahini, and mix well to heat through. Remove from the heat.

FLAVOR BOOST: Serve the stew with chopped fresh parsley or basil.

Per Serving: Calories: 385; Total fat: 23g; Saturated fat: 3g; Sodium: 373mg; Carbohydrates: 27g; Fiber: 7g; Protein: 22g; Calcium: 184mg

Chicken and Orzo Salad

30 MINUTES OR LESS

Serves 4 / Prep time: 10 minutes / Cook time: 15 minutes

Olives, sun-dried tomatoes, and a simple lemon vinaigrette flavor this chicken salad that tastes even better after a day of marinating, making it perfect to pack for weekday lunches or quick dinners. Orzo is typically made from white flour, but using the whole-wheat version makes this a more fiber-rich meal.

1 pound boneless, skinless
  chicken breasts, diced

½ cup Lemon Vinaigrette
  (page 148), divided

1 cup whole-wheat orzo

½ cup chopped sun-dried
  tomatoes

¼ cup chopped
  Kalamata olives

Salt

Freshly ground
  black pepper

1. In a medium bowl, marinate the chicken in ¼ cup of vinaigrette. Let rest for 10 minutes.

2. Meanwhile, fill a large saucepan with water. Bring to a boil.

3. Add the orzo, and cook according to the package directions, or until tender. Remove from the heat. Drain.

4. Meanwhile, heat a large skillet over medium-high heat.

5. Add the chicken and marinade. Cook, stirring regularly, for 5 to 7 minutes, or until cooked through. Remove from the heat.

6. In a large bowl, toss together the chicken, orzo, sun-dried tomatoes, olives, and remaining ¼ cup of vinaigrette. Season with salt and pepper.

FLAVOR BOOST: Serve the salad garnished with ¼ cup of chopped fresh parsley.

Per Serving: Calories: 508; Total fat: 23g; Saturated fat: 3g; Sodium: 406mg; Carbohydrates: 43g; Fiber: 3g; Protein: 30g; Calcium: 37mg

Flank Steak and Hummus Salad

30 MINUTES OR LESS

Serves 4 / Prep time: 15 minutes / Cook time: 15 minutes

Beef should be eaten sparingly, but lean cuts like flank steak are the best choice when you are going to indulge. Cut from the abdominal muscles of the steer, flank steak has more protein and fewer calories than other popular cuts of steak. Be sure to let the beef rest after cooking to allow the juices to redistribute and ensure the finished meat is tender.

1 pound flank steak

Salt

Freshly ground black pepper

8 cups chopped romaine lettuce

½ English cucumber, chopped

½ cup Yogurt-Herb Dressing (page 146), divided

½ cup Garlic Hummus (page 141)

1. Preheat the broiler on high.

2. Season the steak with salt and pepper. Put the steak on a baking sheet.

3. Transfer the baking sheet to the oven, and broil for 5 to 6 minutes. Flip the steak, and broil for 4 to 7 more minutes, depending on your desired doneness. Remove from the oven. Let rest for 10 minutes, then thinly slice against the grain.

4. In a large bowl, toss together the lettuce and cucumber.

5. Drizzle with half of the dressing, and toss again.

6. Serve the salad topped with the steak and hummus.

7. Drizzle with the remaining dressing if desired.

FLAVOR BOOST: Cherry tomatoes and sliced red bell pepper also work really well in this salad.

Per Serving: Calories: 271; Total fat: 12g; Saturated fat: 4g; Sodium: 256mg; Carbohydrates: 13g; Fiber: 3g; Protein: 28g; Calcium: 119mg

Beef Pita Sandwiches

30 MINUTES OR LESS ∘ ONE POT

Serves 4 / Prep time: 5 minutes / Cook time: 15 minutes

In this recipe, lean flank steak is seared on the stovetop, then thinly sliced for a simple pita sandwich that satisfies. The lean cut of beef is best cooked to about medium so that it is nice and tender.

12 ounces flank steak

½ teaspoon garlic powder

½ teaspoon salt

¼ teaspoon freshly ground black pepper

2 tablespoons extra-virgin olive oil

4 whole-wheat pita rounds, halved

½ cup Tahini Dressing (page 145)

1. Season the steak with the garlic powder, salt, and pepper.

2. In a large skillet, heat the oil over medium-high heat.

3. Add the steak, and sear for 5 to 7 minutes per side, or until cooked to your desired doneness. Remove from the heat. Let rest for 5 minutes, then thinly slice against the grain.

4. Stuff several slices of steak into the pita halves.

5. Drizzle with the dressing.

FLAVOR BOOST: Top the sandwiches with lettuce, tomato, and cucumbers to bulk up the vegetable content without adding a lot of calories.

Per Serving: Calories: 377; Total fat: 23g; Saturated fat: 4g; Sodium: 714mg; Carbohydrates: 23g; Fiber: 4g; Protein: 25g; Calcium: 113mg

Chicken and Cauliflower Rice Bowls

30 MINUTES OR LESS ∘ ONE POT

Serves 4 / Prep time: 10 minutes / Cook time: 20 minutes

Cauliflower is a fiber-rich vegetable that is perfect for replacing high-carb items like wheat and rice in your diet. In this bowl, it forms the base and is flavored with the savory goodness of heart-healthy Kalamata olives, which are rich in vitamin E and other antioxidants.

1 pound boneless, skinless chicken breasts, halved lengthwise

½ teaspoon Italian seasoning

½ teaspoon salt

¼ cup freshly ground black pepper

2 tablespoons extra-virgin olive oil, divided

4 cups cauliflower rice

1 (15-ounce) can artichoke hearts, drained

¼ cup chopped Kalamata olives

1. Season the chicken with the Italian seasoning, salt, and pepper.

2. In a large skillet, heat 1 tablespoon of oil over medium-high heat.

3. Add the chicken, and cook for 3 to 5 minutes, or until browned.

4. Flip the chicken, and cook on the other side for 3 to 5 minutes, or until cooked through. Transfer to a cutting board. Thinly slice the chicken across the grain.

5. In the same skillet, heat the remaining 1 tablespoon of oil over medium-high heat.

6. Add the cauliflower rice, and cook for 5 to 8 minutes, or until tender.

7. Add the artichoke hearts and olives. Mix well to heat through. Remove from the heat.

8. Serve the cauliflower and vegetables topped with the chicken.

Per Serving: Calories: 270; Total fat: 11g; Saturated fat: 2g; Sodium: 481mg; Carbohydrates: 14g; Fiber: 6g; Protein: 30g; Calcium: 55mg

Chicken, Quinoa, and Spinach Bowls

30 MINUTES OR LESS

Serves 4 / Prep time: 5 minutes / Cook time: 15 minutes

Quinoa is a whole grain that is rich in fiber, protein, and B vitamins, making it a perfect addition to your heart-healthy meal. The chicken is flavored with za'atar, which pairs wonderfully with the chickpeas and spinach.

2 cups water

1 cup quinoa

1 pound chicken breast tenders

1 teaspoon za'atar

¼ teaspoon salt

¼ teaspoon freshly ground black pepper

2 tablespoons extra-virgin olive oil

1 (15-ounce) can chickpeas, drained and rinsed

4 cups baby spinach

1. In a saucepan, combine the water and quinoa. Bring to a boil.

2. Reduce the heat to a simmer. Cover the saucepan, and cook over low heat for 15 minutes, or until all the water has been absorbed. Remove from the heat.

3. While the quinoa is cooking, season the chicken with the za'atar, salt, and pepper.

4. In a large skillet, heat the oil over medium-high heat.

5. Add the chicken, and sauté for 2 to 3 minutes. Flip, and cook for 3 to 5 minutes, or until browned and cooked through. Remove from the heat.

6. Serve the quinoa topped with the chicken, chickpeas, and spinach.

FLAVOR BOOST: Serve with lemon wedges to squeeze the lemon juice over the bowls.

Per Serving: Calories: 438; Total fat: 14g; Saturated fat: 2g; Sodium: 343mg; Carbohydrates: 41g; Fiber: 7g; Protein: 36g; Calcium: 80mg

Baked Chicken with Tomato, Basil, and Mozzarella

30 MINUTES OR LESS ∘ ONE POT

Serves 4 / Prep time: 5 minutes / Cook time: 25 minutes

Chicken breasts are low in fat and easy to prepare, making them perfect to bake in the oven for a hands-free dish. Serve the chicken breasts over Lemon Rice (page 49) or Zucchini Noodles (page 48) and with a leafy green salad.

1 pound chicken breasts (about 2 breasts), halved lengthwise into 4 pieces

½ teaspoon garlic powder

½ teaspoon salt

¼ teaspoon freshly ground black pepper

½ cup fresh basil leaves

4 mozzarella cheese slices

2 large tomatoes, finely chopped

1. Preheat the oven to 400°F.

2. Season the chicken with the garlic powder, salt, and pepper.

3. Put the chicken on a baking sheet.

4. Transfer the baking sheet to the oven, and bake for 18 to 22 minutes, or until the chicken has cooked through and the juices run clear. Remove from the oven, leaving the oven on.

5. Set the oven to broil on high.

6. Evenly distribute the basil on top of the chicken.

7. Place 1 cheese slice on each breast.

8. Top with the tomatoes.

9. Return the baking sheet to the oven, and broil for 2 to 3 minutes, or until the cheese has melted and browned and the tomatoes are heated through. Remove from the oven.

FLAVOR BOOST: Add ½ teaspoon of Italian seasoning when seasoning the chicken, and serve with lemon wedges.

Per Serving: Calories: 239; Total fat: 9g; Saturated fat: 4g; Sodium: 524mg; Carbohydrates: 4g; Fiber: 1g; Protein: 33g; Calcium: 158mg

Chicken and Artichoke Skillet

ONE POT

Serves 4 / Prep time: 10 minutes / Cook time: 30 minutes

Chicken thighs are a fattier cut of meat than breasts, but that doesn't mean they need to be avoided altogether. Remove the skin first to cut the amount of fat significantly and make them more heart healthy, without losing any of the thigh's juiciness.

2 tablespoons extra-virgin olive oil

4 bone-in chicken thighs, skin removed

¾ teaspoon salt, divided

½ teaspoon freshly ground black pepper, divided

1 (15-ounce) can low-sodium diced tomatoes, drained

¼ cup water

1 (15-ounce) can quartered artichoke hearts, drained

¼ cup pitted Kalamata olives

¼ cup chopped fresh parsley

1. Preheat the oven to 350°F.

2. In a large oven-safe skillet, heat the oil over medium-high heat.

3. Season the chicken with ¼ teaspoon of salt and ¼ teaspoon of pepper. Add to the skillet, and cook for 2 to 3 minutes per side, or until browned. Transfer to a plate.

4. Stir the tomatoes and water into the skillet, and deglaze by scraping up any browned bits from the bottom.

5. Add the artichoke hearts, olives, remaining ½ teaspoon of salt, and ¼ teaspoon of pepper. Mix to combine.

6. Nestle the chicken into the skillet. Turn off the heat.

7. Transfer the skillet to the oven, and bake for 20 minutes, or until the chicken has cooked through. Remove from the oven.

8. Top with the parsley.

MAKE IT EASIER: If you are in a hurry, you can skip the browning step and just combine the ingredients in a baking pan and bake for 30 minutes, or until the chicken has cooked through.

Per Serving: Calories: 270; Total fat: 13g; Saturated fat: 2g; Sodium: 514mg; Carbohydrates: 15g; Fiber: 10g; Protein: 26g; Calcium: 74mg

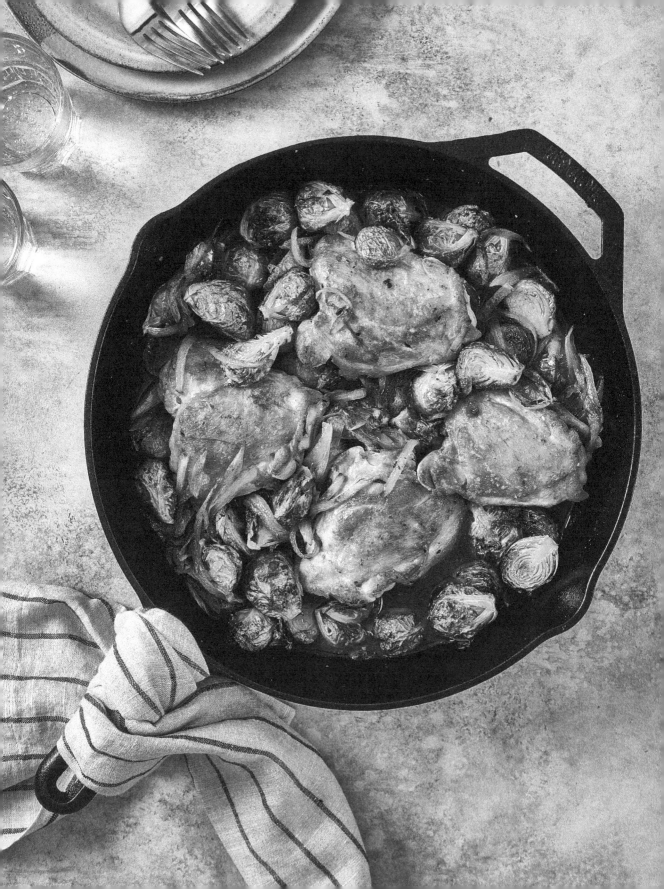

Chicken and Brussels Sprouts Skillet

30 MINUTES OR LESS ∘ ONE POT

Serves 4 / Prep time: 5 minutes / Cook time: 25 minutes

This one-skillet meal starts with searing the chicken on the stove, then finishes off in the oven as the Brussels sprouts tenderize and cook down. If you didn't make the vegetable stock yourself, be sure to buy a low-sodium version to keep the sodium in check.

4 bone-in chicken thighs, skin removed

½ teaspoon salt, divided

¼ teaspoon freshly ground black pepper

2 tablespoons extra-virgin olive oil

1 onion, cut into half-moons

1 pound Brussels sprouts, trimmed and halved

1 cup Vegetable Stock (page 150) or store-bought low-sodium vegetable broth

Juice of 1 lemon

1. Preheat the oven to 350°F.

2. Season the chicken with ½ teaspoon of salt and the pepper.

3. In a large oven-safe skillet, heat the oil over medium-high heat.

4. Place the chicken in the skillet so that the side that had skin faces the bottom, and sear for 3 to 5 minutes, or until browned, then flip.

5. Scatter the onion and Brussels sprouts around the chicken.

6. Add the stock, and bring to a simmer. Turn off the heat.

7. Transfer the skillet to the oven, and bake for 20 minutes, or until cooked through. Remove from the oven.

8. Sprinkle the lemon juice over the top of the chicken and Brussels sprouts.

Per Serving: Calories: 275; Total fat: 12g; Saturated fat: 2g; Sodium: 434mg; Carbohydrates: 17g; Fiber: 5g; Protein: 27g; Calcium: 73mg

Chicken Souvlaki Kebabs

Serves 4 / Prep time: 10 minutes + 30 minutes to rest / Cook time: 15 minutes

This Greek fast-food favorite consists of bite-size marinated pieces of meat cooked on skewers. The tasty meat can be served on its own, over Lemon Rice (page 49), or stuffed into a pita for an easy sandwich. Serve with salad greens, sliced red onions, tomatoes, and cucumber.

1 pound boneless, skinless chicken breasts, cut into 1-inch dice

Juice of 1 lemon

2 tablespoons extra-virgin olive oil

5 garlic cloves, minced

1 teaspoon dried rosemary

1 teaspoon dried oregano

½ teaspoon salt

¼ teaspoon freshly ground black pepper

1. In a medium bowl, combine the chicken, lemon juice, oil, garlic, rosemary, oregano, salt, and pepper. Let rest for 30 minutes.

2. Thread the chicken pieces onto 8 skewers.

3. Preheat a grill on medium-high heat, or preheat a grill pan over medium-high heat.

4. Put the skewers on the grill, and cook for 5 to 7 minutes. Flip, and cook for 5 to 8 minutes, or until cooked through and browned. Remove from the heat.

FLAVOR BOOST: Serve the kebabs with Tzatziki (page 140).

Per Serving: Calories: 205; Total fat: 10g; Saturated fat: 2g; Sodium: 343mg; Carbohydrates: 2g; Fiber: 0g; Protein: 26g; Calcium: 18mg

Chicken Cacciatore

ONE POT

Serves 4 / Prep time: 10 minutes / Cook time: 35 minutes

This one-pot chicken cacciatore is an easy version of the classic dish. Serve it over Zucchini Noodles (page 48) or whole-wheat noodles and with a leafy green salad. Making your own marinara sauce can help keep the sodium in the recipe low, but feel free to substitute a low-sodium store-bought variety to make this dish quickly on a weeknight.

2 tablespoons extra-virgin olive oil

4 bone-in chicken thighs, skin removed

¼ teaspoon salt

¼ teaspoon freshly ground black pepper

1 large onion, sliced

1 red bell pepper, cored and sliced

1 recipe Marinara Sauce (page 143)

1. In a large skillet, heat the oil over medium-high heat.

2. Season the chicken with the salt and pepper. Add the chicken to the skillet, and brown for 2 to 3 minutes per side. Transfer the chicken to a plate.

3. Add the onion and bell pepper to the skillet. Cook for 3 to 5 minutes, or until softened.

4. Add the marinara sauce, and mix well. Bring to a simmer.

5. Return the chicken to the skillet, and simmer for 20 minutes, or until cooked through. Remove from the heat.

FLAVOR BOOST: Garnish the chicken with 2 tablespoons of chopped fresh parsley or cilantro.

Per Serving: Calories: 325; Total fat: 20g; Saturated fat: 4g; Sodium: 482mg; Carbohydrates: 16g; Fiber: 5g; Protein: 25g; Calcium: 93mg

Penne with Pesto, Chicken, and Asparagus

30 MINUTES OR LESS

Serves 4 / Prep time: 5 minutes / Cook time: 15 minutes

Pesto pairs well with chicken to make a quick meal that tastes great. This dish can be made in advance and reheated throughout the week for easy meal prep on busy days. Asparagus increases the nutrition because it's rich in bioflavonoids that help strengthen the immune system, making it a perfect addition to your table.

8 ounces penne

8 ounces boneless, skinless chicken breast, thinly sliced

Salt

Freshly ground black pepper

2 tablespoons extra-virgin olive oil, divided

2 cups chopped asparagus

½ cup Basil-Walnut Pesto (page 144) or store-bought pesto

¼ cup shredded Parmesan cheese

1. Fill a large saucepan with water. Bring to a boil.

2. Cook the penne according to the package directions, until al dente. Remove from the heat. Drain.

3. Meanwhile, season the chicken with salt and pepper.

4. In a large skillet, heat 1 tablespoon of oil over medium-high heat.

5. Add the chicken, and sauté for 5 to 7 minutes, or until cooked through. Transfer the chicken to a plate.

6. In the same skillet, heat the remaining 1 tablespoon of oil over medium-high heat.

7. Add the asparagus, and sauté for 3 to 5 minutes, or until fork tender.

8. Add the chicken, penne, and pesto to the skillet. Mix to combine. Remove from the heat. Season with salt and pepper.

9. Serve topped with the cheese.

SUBSTITUTION TIP: To make this vegetarian, replace the chicken with tofu. Drain 1 (16-ounce) container tofu, and press for 30 minutes between paper towels. Cut into small pieces, and heat the oil over medium-high heat. Pan-fry the pieces of tofu for 3 to 4 minutes, or until lightly browned.

Per Serving: Calories: 543; Total fat: 27g; Saturated fat: 5g; Sodium: 461mg; Carbohydrates: 47g; Fiber: 4g; Protein: 26g; Calcium: 157mg

Pesto Chicken Pizza

Serves 4 / Prep time: 10 minutes / Cook time: 20 minutes

Pizza can be an occasional treat, especially when lightened up with chicken in place of heavily processed meats such as pepperoni and sausage. In this version, we use a store-bought pizza dough for convenience, but if you have a favorite whole-grain pizza dough recipe, substitute it here.

1 premade pizza dough

1 tablespoon extra-virgin olive oil

⅓ cup Basil-Walnut Pesto (page 144)

1 cup shredded cooked chicken

½ cup chopped artichoke hearts

4 ounces fresh mozzarella cheese, thinly sliced

1. Preheat the oven to 425°F.

2. Spread the dough into a thin crust on a large baking sheet or pizza stone, then poke it several times using a fork.

3. Brush the dough with the oil.

4. Transfer the baking sheet to the oven, and bake for 7 minutes, or until the dough has lightly browned. Remove from the oven, leaving the oven on.

5. Spread the pesto on the dough in an even layer to within about ½ inch of the edges.

6. Spread the chicken and artichokes out evenly over the pizza.

7. Top with the cheese.

8. Return the baking sheet to the oven, and bake for 7 to 10 minutes, or until the cheese has melted and browned. Remove from the oven.

Per Serving: Calories: 564; Total fat: 26g; Saturated fat: 7g; Sodium: 623mg; Carbohydrates: 57g; Fiber: 5g; Protein: 28g; Calcium: 222mg

Turkey Burgers

Serves 4 / Prep time: 10 minutes / Cook time: 10 minutes

If you love a good burger, this is going to be a hit. Mild-flavored ground turkey combines with fragrant basil and rich feta to create this hearty Mediterranean-style burger. Serve the burgers on whole-wheat buns or with a large leafy green salad.

1 pound ground turkey

¼ cup crumbled feta cheese

2 tablespoons chopped fresh basil leaves

1 large egg

1 teaspoon Worcestershire sauce

¼ teaspoon freshly ground black pepper

1. In a large bowl, combine the turkey, cheese, basil, egg, Worcestershire sauce, and pepper. Mix well, and form into 4 patties. Transfer to a plate.

2. Heat a large nonstick skillet over medium-high heat.

3. Add the patties, and cook for 3 to 4 minutes per side, or until browned and cooked through. Remove from the heat. Serve with your favorite burger toppings.

SUBSTITUTION TIP: This combination of feta and basil also pairs really nicely in a lamb burger. To make this with lamb, leave out the egg and Worcestershire sauce, and follow the recipe as directed.

Per Serving: Calories: 214; Total fat: 13g; Saturated fat: 4g; Sodium: 196mg; Carbohydrates: 1g; Fiber: 0g; Protein: 24g; Calcium: 81mg

Braised Beef

ONE POT

Serves 6 / Prep time: 10 minutes / Cook time: 1 hour 15 minutes

Braised beef is tender and flavorful with the moisture locked in through the low and slow cooking process. Although beef can be fatty, in a recipe like this, much of the rendered fat can be skimmed off the top, making it a more heart-healthy option. Serve the beef over Polenta Cakes (page 42), cauliflower rice, or Zucchini Noodles (page 48).

1 tablespoon extra-virgin olive oil

1 onion, sliced

3 garlic cloves, minced

1½ pounds beef chuck roast, cut into 1-inch pieces

1 (28-ounce) can whole tomatoes

½ teaspoon freshly ground black pepper

¼ cup chopped fresh parsley

1. Preheat the oven to 350°F.

2. In a large oven-safe pot, heat the oil over medium-high heat.

3. Add the onion, and cook for 3 to 5 minutes, or until slightly softened.

4. Add the garlic, and cook for 30 seconds, or until fragrant.

5. Add the roast, and cook for 5 to 6 minutes, browning it on all sides.

6. Add the tomatoes with their juices, salt, and pepper. Bring to a boil. Turn off the heat.

7. Cover the pot with a lid, and transfer to the oven. Cook, stirring occasionally and scraping up the browned bits off the bottom of the pot, for 1 hour, or until the meat is tender. Remove from the oven. Let rest for 10 minutes.

8. Using a large spoon, skim any fat from the top of the mixture.

9. Serve the roast topped with the parsley.

MAKE IT EASIER: Any braised beef dish like this is going to taste better the next day, and chilling it makes it easier to skim the fat. Once cool, the fat will solidify on top, making it easy to remove.

Per Serving: Calories: 202; Total fat: 9g; Saturated fat: 2g; Sodium: 460mg; Carbohydrates: 7g; Fiber: 3g; Protein: 25g; Calcium: 76mg

Pork and Couscous Skillet

Serves 4 / Prep time: 10 minutes / Cook time: 25 minutes

Thick-cut pork chops will stay moist after cooking in this simple one-pot dish, so opt for them over thinner varieties. Pork chops vary in fattiness, but trimming away the excess fat before cooking can reduce the overall fat content considerably, making them better for heart health.

2 tablespoons extra-virgin olive oil

4 thick-cut pork chops, trimmed

½ onion, chopped

1½ cups Israeli couscous

2½ cups water

½ cup chopped sun-dried tomatoes

3 cups chopped spinach

1. In a large skillet, heat the oil over medium-high heat.

2. Add the pork chops, and brown on both sides for about 1½ minutes per side. Transfer to a plate.

3. Reduce the heat to medium. Add the onion to the skillet, and cook for 3 to 5 minutes, or until softened.

4. Add the couscous, and brown for 1 to 2 minutes.

5. Add the water, and deglaze the skillet by scraping up any browned bits on the bottom.

6. Add the sun-dried tomatoes, and bring to a simmer. Cook for 5 minutes.

7. Return the pork chops to the skillet.

8. Cover the skillet, and reduce the heat to medium-low. Cook for 6 to 8 minutes, or until the pork chops have cooked through and the couscous is tender. If the couscous dries out during cooking, add a splash or two more water to keep it moist. Remove from the heat.

9. Stir in the spinach until wilted.

FLAVOR BOOST: Add ¼ cup of shredded Parmesan cheese to the skillet at the end of cooking with the spinach.

Per Serving: Calories: 484; Total fat: 18g; Saturated fat: 4g; Sodium: 103mg; Carbohydrates: 48g; Fiber: 4g; Protein: 32g; Calcium: 67mg

Herb-Crusted Pork Tenderloin

Serves 6 / Prep time: 5 minutes / Cook time: 30 minutes

Pork tenderloin is a lean cut of meat, making it a perfect option on a heart-healthy diet. Garlic, thyme, cumin, and onion powder combine to season the meat and create a flavorful blend that allows you to go light on salt. Serve with Quinoa Tabbouleh (page 50).

1 teaspoon dried thyme

½ teaspoon ground cumin

½ teaspoon onion powder

¼ teaspoon salt

¼ teaspoon freshly ground black pepper

1½ pounds pork tenderloin

1 tablespoon extra-virgin olive oil

3 garlic cloves, minced

1. Preheat the oven to 400°F.

2. In a small bowl, combine the thyme, cumin, onion powder, salt, and pepper. Mix well.

3. Press the mixture into the pork tenderloin on all sides.

4. In an oven-safe skillet, heat the oil over medium-high heat.

5. Add the garlic, and cook for 30 seconds, or until fragrant.

6. Add the pork, and brown on all sides for 2 to 3 minutes per side. Turn off the heat.

7. Transfer the skillet to the oven, and cook for 15 to 20 minutes, depending on the thickness, or until the pork has cooked through. Remove from the oven.

MAKE IT EASIER: If you have an instant-read thermometer, cooking pork is an excellent time to use it. Pork cuts such as tenderloin, chops, and roasts should all be cooked to 145°F, which is hard to determine just by looking.

Per Serving: Calories: 160; Total fat: 6g; Saturated fat: 2g; Sodium: 157mg; Carbohydrates: 1g; Fiber: 0g; Protein: 24g; Calcium: 13mg

Lamb Kebabs

30 MINUTES OR LESS

Serves 8 / Prep time: 15 minutes / Cook time: 15 minutes

Lamb is a great meat for grilling that benefits wonderfully from the smoky flavor of the grill, where additional fat renders and drips away as it cooks. If you are cooking indoors, use a grill pan for the same effect. Serve the kebabs on pita with Tzatziki (page 140) or Tahini Dressing (page 145).

1 pound ground lamb

1 small onion, chopped

2 tablespoons chopped fresh mint leaves

1 teaspoon ground cumin

1 teaspoon ground coriander

½ teaspoon salt

¼ teaspoon freshly ground black pepper

1.   In a bowl, combine the lamb, onion, mint, cumin, coriander, salt, and pepper. Mix well.

2.   Divide the mixture into 4 pieces. Using wet hands, shape around 8 skewers.

3.   Preheat a grill on medium-high heat, or preheat a grill pan over medium-high heat. (If using a grill pan, also preheat the oven to 400°F.)

4.   Put the kebabs on the grill, and cook on all sides for 2 to 3 minutes per side, or until browned.

5.   Close the lid, and cook for 3 to 5 more minutes, or until the lamb has cooked through. (If using a grill pan, turn off the heat. Put the kebabs on a baking sheet. Transfer the baking sheet to the oven, and bake for 3 to 5 minutes.) Remove from the heat.

SUBSTITUTION TIP: This recipe can be made using lean ground beef instead.

Per Serving: Calories: 247; Total fat: 20g; Saturated fat: 9g; Sodium: 269mg; Carbohydrates: 1g; Fiber: 0g; Protein: 14g; Calcium: 20mg

Ras el Hanout Lamb Stew

Serves 4 / Prep time: 5 minutes / Cook time: 50 minutes

Lamb benefits from stewing to make it tender and fall-apart perfect. This protein-packed stew is hearty and warming with the inclusion of ras el hanout, a blend of spices that typically includes cinnamon, nutmeg, clove, cumin, cardamom, allspice, chile peppers, and more. If you don't have it, you can make a simple substitution using 1 teaspoon paprika, 1 teaspoon coriander, and ½ teaspoon ground ginger.

2 tablespoons extra-virgin olive oil

1 pound boneless lamb shoulder (stew meat), diced

1 large onion, chopped

2 carrots, chopped

1 (15-ounce) can chickpeas, drained and rinsed

2 teaspoons ras el hanout

4 cups water

½ teaspoon salt

¼ teaspoon freshly ground black pepper

1. In a large pot, heat the oil over medium-high heat.

2. Add the lamb, and brown on all sides for 3 to 5 minutes per side. Leaving the juices in the pot, transfer the lamb to a plate.

3. Add the onion and carrots to the pot. Cook for 3 to 5 minutes, or until softened and browned.

4. Add the chickpeas and ras el hanout. Mix well.

5. Add the lamb back to the pot, along with any juices that have collected on the plate. Add the water, and bring to a boil.

6. Reduce the heat to low. Cover the pot, and simmer for 30 to 40 minutes, or until the lamb is tender. Remove from the heat. Season with the salt and pepper.

Per Serving: Calories: 399; Total fat: 25g; Saturated fat: 8g; Sodium: 501mg; Carbohydrates: 20g; Fiber: 5g; Protein: 26g; Calcium: 55mg

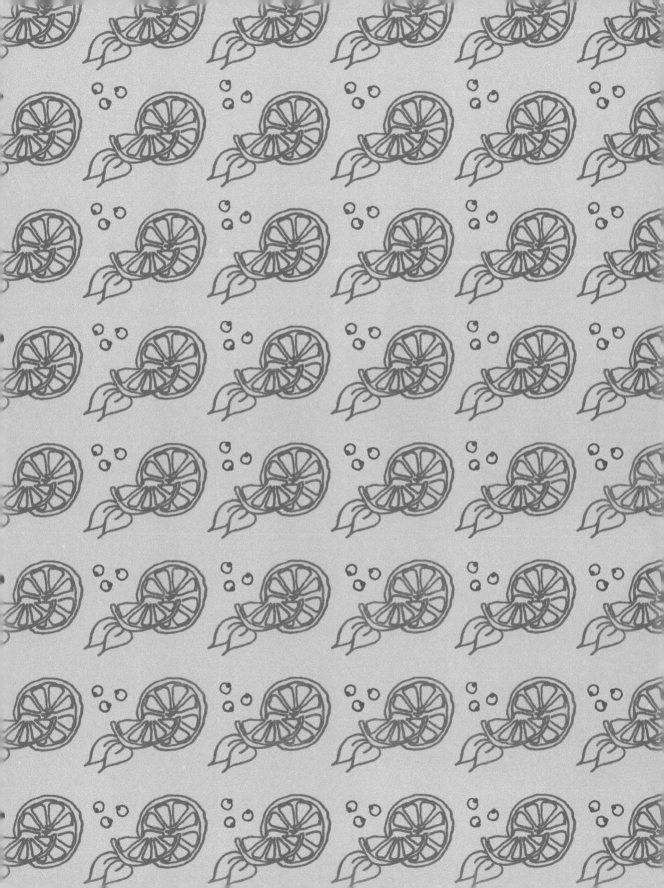

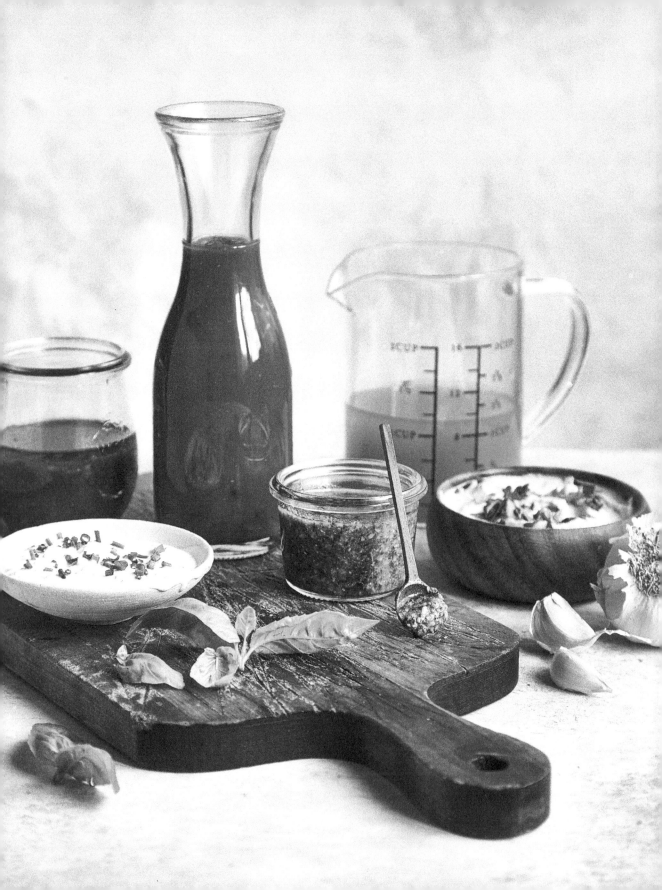

CHAPTER SEVEN

Sauces, Staples, and Sweet Treats

Tzatziki

This classic yogurt sauce is fresh and minty and loaded with cucumber. To prevent the sauce from being runny, be sure not to skip the step of wringing out the cucumber. Greek yogurt is loaded with protein and probiotics, making it a healthy sauce to use regularly to flavor dishes and provide a cool, refreshing contrast to warm, savory dishes. The Chickpea Gyros (page 67) and Portabella Mushroom Gyros (page 68) both use it for this purpose.

1 cucumber, peeled and grated

1½ cups plain, unsweetened, low-fat Greek yogurt

1 tablespoon extra-virgin olive oil

1 tablespoon freshly squeezed lemon juice

1 tablespoon chopped fresh mint leaves

2 garlic cloves, minced

½ teaspoon salt

1. Working over the sink, squeeze the cucumber in batches, extracting as much water as possible. Put the cucumber in a bowl.

2. Add the yogurt, oil, lemon juice, mint, garlic, and salt. Mix well. Let rest for 10 minutes before serving.

SUBSTITUTION TIP: If you avoid dairy, use unsweetened coconut yogurt in place of the Greek yogurt.

Per Serving (¼ cup): Calories: 48; Total fat: 2g; Saturated fat: 1g; Sodium: 178mg; Carbohydrates: 4g; Fiber: 0g; Protein: 3g; Calcium: 89mg

Garlic Hummus

Makes 1¼ cups / Prep time: 10 minutes

A can of chickpeas can be transformed into a batch of delicious hummus in just minutes. Hummus is rich in protein and fiber, making it a great snack option and perfect for spreading on your favorite sandwiches and for dipping vegetables. Hummus can be stored for up to 5 days, so make a batch at the beginning of the week to have on hand throughout the week. It adds protein and great flavor to Fried Eggplant, Zucchini, and Tomatoes (page 82) and Flank Steak and Hummus Salad (page 114).

1 (15-ounce) can low-sodium chickpeas, drained and rinsed

Juice of 1 lemon

2 tablespoons tahini

3 garlic cloves, peeled

½ teaspoon salt

2 tablespoons extra-virgin olive oil

2 tablespoons chopped fresh parsley

1. In a blender or food processor, combine the chickpeas, lemon juice, tahini, garlic, and salt. Process until combined.

2. With the blender running, stream in the oil, and continue blending until smooth.

3. Serve the hummus topped with the parsley.

FLAVOR BOOST: Sprinkle paprika and drizzle a little olive oil on top of the hummus.

Per Serving (2 tablespoons): Calories: 76; Total fat: 5g; Saturated fat: 1g; Sodium: 129mg; Carbohydrates: 7g; Fiber: 2g; Protein: 2g; Calcium: 26mg

Baba Ghanoush

VEGAN ○ VEGETARIAN

Makes about 1¼ cups / Prep time: 10 minutes / Cook time: 30 minutes

The smoky cousin of hummus, baba ghanoush is a similarly savory dip made from roasted eggplant, tahini, and olive oil. Often served with pita bread, baba ghanoush is also a great sandwich spread and dip for veggies. It is a low-fat, heart-healthy alternative to cream and cheese dips and spreads.

1 large globe eggplant

2 tablespoons tahini

Juice of 1 lemon

2 garlic cloves, peeled

2 tablespoons extra-virgin olive oil

½ teaspoon ground cumin

1. Preheat the oven to 350°F.

2. Using a fork, poke holes in the eggplant 2 or 3 times.

3. Put the eggplant on a baking sheet.

4. Transfer the baking sheet to the oven, and bake for 25 to 30 minutes, or until the eggplant has softened. Remove from the oven. Let cool.

5. Once cool enough to handle, peel the skin off the eggplant, and put the flesh in a blender.

6. Add the tahini, lemon juice, garlic, oil, and cumin. Process until smooth, adding 1 or 2 tablespoons of water as needed.

FLAVOR BOOST: Sprinkle with regular or smoked paprika.

Per Serving (2 tablespoons): Calories: 58; Total fat: 4g; Saturated fat: 1g; Sodium: 5mg; Carbohydrates: 4g; Fiber: 2g; Protein: 1g; Calcium: 20mg

Marinara Sauce

30 MINUTES OR LESS ○ ONE POT ○ VEGAN ○ VEGETARIAN

Makes about 2 cups / Prep time: 5 minutes / Cook time: 20 minutes

This is an easy go-to sauce that you can prepare in a matter of minutes and makes dishes like Chicken Cacciatore (page 125) shine. Whole tomatoes have the most flavor; break them up with a spoon as you go, and by the time the sauce cooks down a bit, you will have a nice chunky marinara sauce. If you want a smoother sauce, use an immersion blender to puree it.

2 tablespoons extra-virgin olive oil

1 onion, chopped

2 garlic cloves, minced

1 (28-ounce) can whole tomatoes

1 thyme sprig

2 tablespoons chopped fresh basil leaves

1. In a large saucepan, heat the oil over medium-high heat.

2. Add the onion, and sauté for 3 to 5 minutes, or until softened and lightly browned.

3. Add the garlic, and cook for 30 seconds, or until fragrant.

4. Add the tomatoes with their juices, breaking them up using a spoon as you mix.

5. Add the thyme, and simmer for 10 minutes, or until the flavors meld. Remove from the heat.

6. Top with the basil.

FLAVOR BOOST: Add a pinch red pepper flakes for a spicy marinara.

Per Serving (¼ cup): Calories: 52; Total fat: 4g; Saturated fat: 1g; Sodium: 115mg; Carbohydrates: 5g; Fiber: 2g; Protein: 1g; Calcium: 38mg

Basil-Walnut Pesto

30 MINUTES OR LESS ○ ONE POT

Makes about 1 cup / Prep time: 10 minutes

This easy herbal sauce is traditionally made with basil, pine nuts, garlic, and olive oil, but here walnuts are used in place of the pine nuts. They are much less expensive than pine nuts and are the only nut that is an excellent source of omega-3s, making them a great choice for a heart-healthy diet.

2 cups packed basil leaves

¼ cup chopped walnuts

¼ cup shredded
 Parmesan cheese

3 garlic cloves, peeled

½ teaspoon salt

¼ cup extra-virgin olive oil

1. In a food processor, combine the basil, walnuts, cheese, garlic, and salt. Pulse several times until broken into small pieces.

2. With the food processor running, stream in the oil until smooth.

SUBSTITUTION TIP: If you don't have basil, use kale in its place for a milder yet equally delicious flavor.

Per Serving (2 tablespoons): Calories: 100; Total fat: 10g; Saturated fat: 2g; Sodium: 202mg; Carbohydrates: 1g; Fiber: 0g; Protein: 2g; Calcium: 43mg

Tahini Dressing

30 MINUTES OR LESS ○ ONE POT ○ VEGAN ○ VEGETARIAN

Makes ½ cup / Prep time: 10 minutes

Tahini has a distinctive nutty flavor that lends itself well to a dressing. Whether you drizzle it on a pita sandwich, a salad, or a Tahini and Black Bean–Stuffed Sweet Potato (page 64), this easy dressing is sure to top it well. Sesame seeds are a good source of fiber and plant protein, making them a heart-healthy choice.

⅓ cup tahini

Juice of 1 lemon

1 teaspoon maple syrup

2 garlic cloves, minced

½ teaspoon salt

¼ teaspoon freshly ground black pepper

In a bowl, whisk together the tahini, lemon juice, maple syrup, garlic, salt, and pepper. Add 2 to 3 tablespoons of water as needed to create a smooth dressing.

MAKE IT EASIER: Make this dressing up to 5 days in advance, and store in an airtight container in the refrigerator.

Per Serving (2 tablespoons): Calories: 127; Total fat: 11g; Saturated fat: 1g; Sodium: 314mg; Carbohydrates: 7g; Fiber: 2g; Protein: 4g; Calcium: 90mg

Yogurt-Herb Dressing

30 MINUTES OR LESS ○ ONE POT ○ VEGETARIAN

Makes 1¼ cups / Prep time: 10 minutes

Creamy dressings don't have to be ditched as part of your heart-healthy eating plan, but they do need to be reworked with healthier ingredients. Low-fat yogurt shines in this simple herby dressing that is a good alternative to creamy mayonnaise-based dressings.

1 cup plain, unsweetened, low-fat Greek yogurt

¼ cup chopped fresh chives

¼ cup chopped fresh parsley

2 tablespoons extra-virgin olive oil

2 tablespoons rice vinegar

2 garlic cloves, minced

¼ teaspoon salt

¼ teaspoon freshly ground black pepper

In a small bowl, whisk together the yogurt, chives, parsley, oil, vinegar, garlic, salt, and pepper to combine. Store in an airtight container in the refrigerator for up to 5 days.

SUBSTITUTION TIP: Use 1 tablespoon of dried chives and 1 tablespoon of dried parsley in place of the fresh.

Per Serving (2 tablespoons): Calories: 42; Total fat: 3g; Saturated fat: 1g; Sodium: 76mg; Carbohydrates: 2g; Fiber: 0g; Protein: 1g; Calcium: 49mg

Balsamic Vinaigrette

30 MINUTES OR LESS ◦ ONE POT ◦ VEGAN ◦ VEGETARIAN

Makes ¾ cup / Prep time: 5 minutes

Having a simple and delicious balsamic vinaigrette will provide you with an easy go-to dressing when you need to make a quick salad. Skip store-bought salad dressings, which are full of inexpensive oils that don't promote good health, and make this vinaigrette with heart-healthy olive oil.

3 tablespoons balsamic vinegar

2 teaspoons Dijon mustard

2 teaspoons maple syrup

1 large garlic clove, minced

¼ teaspoon salt

¼ teaspoon freshly ground black pepper

½ cup extra-virgin olive oil

2 tablespoons chopped fresh thyme leaves

1. In a small bowl or jar, whisk together the vinegar, mustard, maple syrup, garlic, salt, and pepper.

2. While whisking, stream in the oil until emulsified.

3. Stir in the thyme. Cover, and refrigerate for up to 5 days.

FLAVOR BOOST: Add a minced shallot to the dressing.

Per Serving (2 tablespoons): Calories: 174; Total fat: 18g; Saturated fat: 2g; Sodium: 118mg; Carbohydrates: 3g; Fiber: 0g; Protein: 0g; Calcium: 10mg

Lemon Vinaigrette

30 MINUTES OR LESS ◦ ONE POT ◦ VEGAN ◦ VEGETARIAN

Makes about ¾ cup / Prep time: 10 minutes

The brightness of lemon is a perfect pairing with salads and proteins, making this a great dressing to have on hand. Lemon is loaded with vitamin C, a powerful antioxidant that protects cells from free-radical damage, and it is a wonderful ingredient to give a variety of dishes bright, distinctive flavor.

Juice of 2 lemons

Zest of 1 lemon

1 tablespoon Dijon mustard

2 garlic cloves, minced

2 teaspoons maple syrup

1 teaspoon fresh thyme leaves

½ teaspoon salt

½ teaspoon freshly ground black pepper

½ cup extra-virgin olive oil

1. In a small bowl, whisk together the lemon juice, lemon zest, mustard, garlic, maple syrup, thyme, salt, and pepper.

2. Stream in the oil, and whisk until emulsified.

SUBSTITUTION TIP: This same recipe can be used with lime or orange in place of the lemon. You will need to use 3 or 4 limes or 1 large orange to get ¼ cup of juice.

Per Serving (2 tablespoons): Calories: 172; Total fat: 18g; Saturated fat: 2g; Sodium: 223mg; Carbohydrates: 3g; Fiber: 0g; Protein: 0g; Calcium: 7mg

Yogurt-Tahini Dip

30 MINUTES OR LESS ○ ONE POT ○ VEGETARIAN

Makes 1¼ cups / Prep time: 10 minutes + 1 hour to chill

Tahini, a paste made from ground sesame seeds, is a flavorful ingredient that adds a creamy richness to this yogurt-based dip. Look for tahini with other nut butters or in the international section of your supermarket. Serve the dip with Vegetable Chips with Rosemary Salt (page 33), Roasted Sweet Potato Fries (page 40), or cut vegetables such as cucumbers, carrots, bell peppers, or cauliflower.

1 cup plain, unsweetened, low-fat Greek yogurt

3 tablespoons tahini

Juice of 1 lemon

1 large garlic clove, minced

1 teaspoon za'atar

Salt

Freshly ground black pepper

In a small bowl, mix together the yogurt, tahini, lemon juice, garlic, and za'atar. Season with salt and pepper. Refrigerate for at least 1 hour before serving.

FLAVOR BOOST: Add ½ teaspoon of ground cumin, and top with 3 tablespoons of chopped fresh cilantro.

Per Serving (¼ cup): Calories: 87; Total fat: 6g; Saturated fat: 1g; Sodium: 76mg; Carbohydrates: 6g; Fiber: 1g; Protein: 4g; Calcium: 130mg

Vegetable Stock

VEGAN ○ VEGETARIAN

Makes about 8 cups / Prep time: 5 minutes / Cook time: 1 hour

When you make stock on your own, the finished product has a lot less sodium than store-bought varieties. Although this stock uses whole vegetables, you can also use vegetable scraps and peels in their place. Save up onion, carrot, celery, and mushroom trimmings in a resealable bag in the freezer until you have the same amount of scraps as whole vegetables. Enjoy this in Minestrone (page 56) and Egg, Lemon, and Chicken Soup (page 111).

2 cups mushrooms	2 carrots	4 or 5 thyme sprigs
1 onion	3 celery stalks	8 cups water

1. In a large stockpot, combine the mushrooms, onion, carrots, celery, thyme, and water. Bring to a boil over high heat.

2. Reduce the heat to low. Simmer for 1 hour. Remove from the heat. Strain into a bowl, pressing the vegetables into the strainer using the back of a spoon to extract as much liquid as possible. Let cool to room temperature, then refrigerate for up to 5 days, or freeze for up to 3 months.

MAKE IT EASIER: Freeze the stock in different-size containers so you can thaw only as much as you need. Use an ice cube tray, then transfer the cubes to a freezer-safe bag for sauces, and pint- and quart-size containers for soups and stews.

Per Serving (1 cup): Calories: 10; Total fat: 0g; Saturated fat: 0g; Sodium: 20mg; Carbohydrates: 3g; Fiber: 0g; Protein: 0g; Calcium: 0mg

Honey-Sweetened Yogurt with Balsamic-Mint Berries

30 MINUTES OR LESS ◦ VEGETARIAN

Serves 4 / Prep time: 10 minutes

Yogurt is a powerful probiotic that can double as the centerpiece of dessert. Sweeten the yogurt with honey, and top with berries soaked in balsamic vinegar for a simple treat that hits the spot when your sweet tooth strikes.

2 cups plain, unsweetened, low-fat Greek yogurt

1 tablespoon honey

2 cups mixed fresh berries, such as strawberries, blackberries, blueberries

2 tablespoons balsamic vinegar

2 tablespoons thinly sliced fresh mint

1. In a small bowl, stir together the yogurt and honey to combine.

2. In another small bowl, combine the berries and vinegar. Using a fork, lightly mash. Let rest for a few minutes.

3. Serve the yogurt topped with ½ cup of fruit and ½ tablespoon of the mint.

FLAVOR BOOST: Sprinkle up to ¼ cup of low-sugar granola to each serving to make it more of a parfait.

Per Serving: Calories: 127; Total fat: 2g; Saturated fat: 1g; Sodium: 89mg; Carbohydrates: 21g; Fiber: 2g; Protein: 7g; Calcium: 240mg

Cinnamon Pear Crisp

VEGAN ○ VEGETARIAN

Serves 8 / Prep time: 10 minutes / Cook time: 45 minutes

If you are going to enjoy sweets, whole, natural foods are the best choice for your health. Pears are naturally sweet and, when baked with cinnamon, have an amazing aroma that fills the house. Oats and pears are rich in fiber and antioxidants, making them wonderful building blocks for a heart-healthy dessert.

6 medium pears, cored and cut into ¼-inch-thick slices

4 tablespoons maple syrup, divided

1 teaspoon ground cinnamon

¾ cup rolled oats, divided

½ cup chopped walnuts

3 tablespoons extra-virgin olive oil

1. Preheat the oven to 350°F.

2. In a bowl, combine the pears, 3 tablespoons of maple syrup, and the cinnamon. Mix well.

3. Spread the pears out in an even layer in an 8-inch baking dish.

4. In a food processor or blender, process ¼ cup of oats on high speed until powdered. Transfer to a small bowl.

5. To the oat flour, add the remaining ½ cup of oats and the walnuts. Mix well.

6. Drizzle with the oil and the remaining 1 tablespoon of maple syrup. Toss to coat.

7. Crumble the mixture over the top of the pears in an even layer.

8. Transfer the baking dish to the oven, and bake for 45 minutes, or until the crumble has browned. Remove from the oven.

Per Serving: Calories: 241; Total fat: 11g; Saturated fat: 1g; Sodium: 3mg; Carbohydrates: 36g; Fiber: 6g; Protein: 4g; Calcium: 39mg

Date Brownies

VEGETARIAN

Makes 16 brownies / Prep time: 15 minutes / Cook time: 30 minutes

Most baked goods are loaded with refined grains and sugars, but these brownies use naturally sweet dates and almond flour for a rich alternative to the typical brownie. Dates are full of fiber and antioxidants, making them more protective to the heart than the usual white sugar and a perfect ingredient to sweeten these brownies.

Nonstick cooking spray

2 cups pitted dates

3 large eggs

1 cup almond flour

½ cup cocoa powder

¼ cup avocado oil

1 teaspoon baking soda

Pinch salt

1. Preheat the oven to 350°F. Spray an 8-inch baking dish with cooking spray.

2. Bring a small pot of water to a boil over high heat. Remove from the heat.

3. In a bowl, cover the pitted dates with the boiling water, and let soak for 15 minutes. Drain.

4. In a food processor, combine the dates and 2 tablespoons of water. Process until smooth, adding up to 2 tablespoons more water if needed.

5. Add the eggs, one at a time, mixing between each addition.

6. Add the flour, cocoa powder, oil, baking soda, and salt. Mix again. Transfer to the prepared baking dish.

7. Transfer the baking dish to the oven, and bake for 30 minutes, or until a toothpick inserted into the center of the brownies comes out mostly clean. Remove from the oven. Let cool, then cut into 16 pieces.

Per Serving (1 brownie): Calories: 125; Total fat: 7g; Saturated fat: 1g; Sodium: 103mg; Carbohydrates: 16g; Fiber: 3g; Protein: 3g; Calcium: 27mg

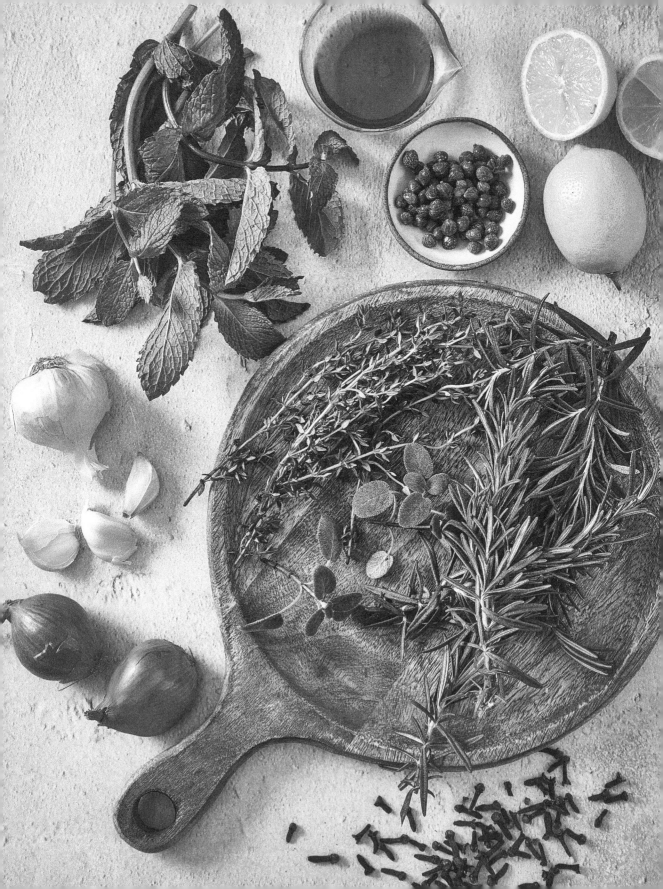

— MEASUREMENT CONVERSIONS —

Volume Equivalents	US STANDARD	US STANDARD (OUNCES)	METRIC (APPROXIMATE)
Liquid	2 tablespoons	1 fl. oz.	30 mL
	¼ cup	2 fl. oz.	60 mL
	½ cup	4 fl. oz.	120 mL
	1 cup	8 fl. oz.	240 mL
	1½ cups	12 fl. oz.	355 mL
	2 cups or 1 pint	16 fl. oz.	475 mL
	4 cups or 1 quart	32 fl. oz.	1 L
	1 gallon	128 fl. oz.	4 L
Dry	⅛ teaspoon	—	0.5 mL
	¼ teaspoon	—	1 mL
	½ teaspoon	—	2 mL
	¾ teaspoon	—	4 mL
	1 teaspoon	—	5 mL
	1 tablespoon	—	15 mL
	¼ cup	—	59 mL
	⅓ cup	—	79 mL
	½ cup	—	118 mL
	⅔ cup	—	156 mL
	¾ cup	—	177 mL
	1 cup	—	235 mL
	2 cups or 1 pint	—	475 mL
	3 cups	—	700 mL
	4 cups or 1 quart	—	1 L
	½ gallon	—	2 L
	1 gallon	—	4 L

Oven Temperatures

FAHRENHEIT	CELSIUS (APPROXIMATE)
250°F	120°C
300°F	150°C
325°F	165°C
350°F	180°C
375°F	190°C
400°F	200°C
425°F	220°C
450°F	230°C

Weight Equivalents

US STANDARD	METRIC (APPROXIMATE)
½ ounce	15 g
1 ounce	30 g
2 ounces	60 g
4 ounces	115 g
8 ounces	225 g
12 ounces	340 g
16 ounces or 1 pound	455 g

— REFERENCES —

Aune, Dagfinn, Edward Giovannucci, Paolo Boffetta, Lars T. Fadnes, NaNa Keum, Teresa Norat, Darren C. Greenwood, Elio Riboli, Lars J. Vatten, and Serena Tonstad. "Fruit and Vegetable Intake and the Risk of Cardiovascular Disease, Total Cancer and All-Cause Mortality–A Systematic Review and Dose-Response Meta-Analysis of Prospective Studies." *International Journal of Epidemiology* 46, no. 3 (June 2017): 1029–56. doi.org/10.1093/ije/dyw319.

Bazzano Lydia A., Jiang He, Lorraine G. Ogden, Catherine Loria, Suma Vupputuri, Leann Myers, and Paul K. Whelton. "Legume Consumption and Risk of Coronary Heart Disease in US Men and Women: NHANES I Epidemiologic Follow-up Study." *Archives of Internal Medicine* 161, no. 21 (2001): 2573–78. doi.org/10.1001/archinte.161.21.2573.

Centers for Disease Control and Prevention. "FastStats—Deaths and Mortality." Last modified November 21, 2020. CDC.gov/nchs/fastats/deaths.htm.

Challa, Hima J., Muhammad Atif Ameer, and Kalyan R. Uppaluri. "DASH Diet to Stop Hypertension." StatPearls Publishing. Last modified May 23, 2020. ncbi.nlm.NIH.gov/books/NBK482514.

DiNicolantonio, James J., and James H. O'Keefe. "Effects of Dietary Fats on Blood Lipids: A Review of Direct Comparison Trials." *Open Heart* 5 (July 2018): e000871. doi.org/10.1136/openhrt-2018-000871.

Estruch, Ramón, Emilio Ros, Jordi Salas-Salvadó, Maria-Isabel Covas, Dolores Corella, Fernando Arós, Enrique Gómez-Gracia, et. al. "Primary Prevention of Cardiovascular Disease with a Mediterranean Diet Supplemented with Extra-Virgin Olive Oil or Nuts." *The New England Journal of Medicine* 378 (June 2018): e34. doi.org/10.1056/nejmoa1800389.

Guasch-Ferré, Marta, Xiaoran Liu, Vasanti S. Malik, Qi Sun, Walter C. Willett, JoAnn E. Manson, Kathryn M. Rexrode, Yanping Li, Frank B. Hu, and Shilpa N. Bhupathiraju. "Nut Consumption and Risk of Cardiovascular Disease." *Journal of the American College of Cardiology* 70, no. 20 (Nov. 2017): 2519–32. doi.org/10.1016/j.jacc.2017.09.035.

Hu, Yang, Frank B. Hu, and JoAnn E. Manson. "Marine Omega-3 Supplementation and Cardiovascular Disease: An Updated Meta-Analysis of 13 Randomized Controlled Trials Involving 127,477 Participants." *Journal of the American Heart Association* 8, no. 19 (October 2019). doi.org/10.1161/jaha.119.013543.

Jenkins, David J.A., Peter J. H. Jones, Benoit Lamarche, Cyril W. C. Kendall, Dorothea Faulkner, Luba Cermakova, and Iris Gigleux. "Effect of a Dietary Portfolio of Cholesterol-Lowering Foods Given at 2 Levels of Intensity of Dietary Advice on Serum Lipids in Hyperlipidemia: A Randomized Controlled Trial." *Journal of the American Medical Association* 306, no. 8 (August 2011): 831–839. doi.org/10.1001/jama.2011.1202.

Khaw, Kay-Tee, Stephen J. Sharp, Leila Finikarides, Islam Afzal, Marleen Lentjes, Robert Luben, and Nita G. Forouhi. "Randomised Trial of Coconut Oil, Olive Oil or Butter on Blood Lipids and Other Cardiovascular Risk Factors in Healthy Men and Women." *British Medical Journal Open* 8, no. 3 (March 2018): e020167. doi.org/10.1136/bmjopen-2017-020167.

Khurana, Sandhya, Krishnan Venkataraman, Amanda Hollingsworth, Matthew Piche, and T. C. Tai. "Polyphenols: Benefits to the Cardiovascular System in Health and in Aging." *Nutrients* 5, no. 10 (October 2013): 3779–3827. doi.org/10.3390/nu5103779.

Lattimer, James M., and Mark D. Haub. "Effects of Dietary Fiber and Its Components on Metabolic Health." *Nutrients* 2, no. 12 (December 2010): 1266–89. doi.org/10.3390/nu2121266.

Liu, Xiaoran, Marta Guasch-Ferré, Jean-Philippe Drouin-Chartier, Deirdre K. Tobias, Shilpa N. Bhupathiraju, Kathryn M. Rexrode, Walter C. Willett, Qi Sun, and Yanping Li. "Changes in Nut Consumption and Subsequent Cardiovascular Disease Risk Among US Men and Women: 3 Large Prospective Cohort Studies." *Journal of the American Heart Association* 9, no. 7 (April 2020). doi.org/10.1161/jaha.119.013877.

Melina, Vesanto, Winston Craig, and Susan Levin. "Position of the Academy of Nutrition and Dietetics: Vegetarian Diets." *Journal of the Academy of Nutrition and Dietetics* 116, no. 12 (December 2016): 1970–80. doi.org/10.1016/j.jand .2016.09.025.

Miller, Victoria, Andrew Mente, Mahshid Dehghan, Sumathy Rangarajan, Xiaohe Zhang, Sumathi Swaminathan, Gilles Dagenais, et al. "Fruit, Vegetable, and Legume Intake, and Cardiovascular Disease and Deaths in 18 Countries (PURE): A Prospective Cohort Study." *The Lancet* 390, no. 10107, (November 2017): 2037–49. doi.org/10.1016/S0140-6736(17)32253-5.

Ramdath, D. Dan, Emily M. T. Padhi, Sidra Sarfaraz, Simone Renwick, and Alison M. Duncan. "Beyond the Cholesterol-Lowering Effect of Soy Protein: A Review of the Effects of Dietary Soy and Its Constituents on Risk Factors for Cardiovascular Disease." *Nutrients* 9, no. 4 (April 2017): 324. doi.org/10.3390/nu9040324.

Staruschenko, Alexander. "Beneficial Effects of High Potassium." *Hypertension* 71, no. 6 (June 2018): 1015–22. doi.org/10.1161/hypertensionaha.118.10267.

Tangney, Christy C., and Heather E. Rasmussen. "Polyphenols, Inflammation, and Cardiovascular Disease." *Current Atherosclerosis Reports* 15 (March 2013): 324. doi.org/10.1007/s11883-013-0324-x.

Yan, Zhaoli, Xinyue Zhang, Chunlin Li, Shouchun Jiao, and Wenyao Dong. "Association between Consumption of Soy and Risk of Cardiovascular Disease: A Meta-Analysis of Observational Studies." *European Journal of Preventive Cardiology* 24, no. 7 (May 2017): 735–747. doi.org/10.1177/2047487316686441.

Zhong, Victor W., Linda Van Horn, Philip Greenland, Mercedes R. Carnethon, Hongyan Ning, John T. Wilkins, Donald M. Lloyd-Jones, and Norrina B. Allen. "Associations of Processed Meat, Unprocessed Red Meat, Poultry, or Fish Intake with Incident Cardiovascular Disease and All-Cause Mortality." *JAMA Internal Medicine* 180, no. 4: 503–12. doi.org/10.1001/jamainternmed.2019.6969.

— INDEX —

Z

Zucchini

Eggs over Sautéed Tomato, Bell
Pepper, and Zucchini, 22

Feta and Black Bean–Stuffed Zucchini, 78–79

Fried Eggplant, Zucchini, and Tomatoes, 82–83

Omelet with Zucchini, Mushrooms,
and Peppers, 23

Roasted Peppers and Zucchini, 41

Vegetable Chips with Rosemary Salt, 33–34

Vegetable Frittata, 24

Zucchini Noodles, 48

— ABOUT THE AUTHOR —

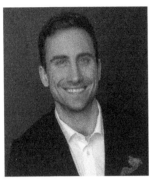

Andy De Santis, RD, MPH, is a registered dietitian, speaker, and three-time author from Toronto, Canada. He operates a private dietetics practice focused on customized nutrition solutions for people dealing with a wide variety of issues and prides himself on providing exceptional care to his clients. Andy has been featured in local newspapers and magazines and on television. He is never afraid to provide his views on topics of importance. When he isn't helping people in a one-on-one setting, Andy loves creating hard-hitting content with a lighthearted twist, which he shares through his personal blog, AndyTheRD.com, and various social media accounts, including Instagram (@AndyTheRD).

— ABOUT THE RECIPE DEVELOPER —

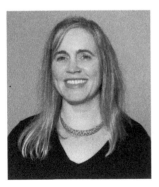

Katherine Green is a cookbook author, editor, and recipe developer living in Portland, Oregon, with her husband and two sons. She is passionate about fermentation, home cooking, and gardening and specializes in creating recipes for specific dietary needs. She has completed a certificate program in nutritional therapy and holds a bachelor's degree in journalism from Western Michigan University.